For Annie Hopcraft with deepest love – I shall miss you.

And for Russell and Chris.

Acknowledgements

The editors wish to thank the Wellcome Foundation for providing funding support for the conference in Birmingham in May 2007, Mickey Willmott for help with the editing, and all the contributors and those who attended the Birmingham conference.

Contents

List of figures, tables and boxes

Figures

Tables

Boxes

Notes on contributors

Jo Abbott works in a busy public health department in an area of high deprivation following the closure of the coal and steel industries across South Yorkshire, UK. Her interests include reducing health inequalities, and access to evidence-based care. Jo's portfolio includes coronary heart disease, R&D, emergency planning (including for pandemic influenza) and health impact assessment. Jo is an accredited trainer for public health trainees and an assessor for specialists in public health wishing to enter the Public Health Specialist Voluntary Register. Jo currently Chairs South Yorkshire Research Ethics Committee.

Peter Allmark is a Principal Lecturer at Sheffield Hallam University, UK. His clinical background is in acute and critical care nursing while his academic background is in philosophy and ethics. He has published extensively in the field of health care ethics. He has worked on a number of research projects, including Euricon and the Toby-Qual study. His current research interests are in ethics, public health and health inequality.

Alan Cribb is Professor of Bioethics and Education and Director of the Centre for Public Policy, King's College London. His research relates to applied philosophy and health policy. He has a particular interest in developing interdisciplinary scholarship that links philosophical, social science and professional concerns, and he has pursued this interest through writing about health care ethics, public health, and health and education policy. His most recent books are *Understanding education* (2009, with Sharon Gewirtz, Cambridge: Polity Press), *Health and the good society* (2008, Oxford: Oxford University Press) and an edited collection on *Nursing law and ethics* (2007, with J. Tingle, Oxford: Blackwell Science).

Jessica Datta is a Research Fellow in the Centre for Sexual and Reproductive Health at the London School of Hygiene & Tropical Medicine. Her research interests include sexual behaviour, the evaluation of public health interventions, and the health and well-being of children and young people.

Angus Dawson is Senior Lecturer in Ethics and Philosophy at the Centre for Professional Ethics, Keele University, UK. His background is in philosophy, although he was worked in applied ethics for over ten years. His main research interests are in public health ethics (particularly vaccinations) and the use of empirical evidence in moral arguments (particularly in relation to problems in gaining informed consent in clinical trials). He is joint co-ordinator of the International Association of Bioethics' Public Health Ethics Network (InterPHEN) with Marcel Verweij. He has published numerous papers and book chapters and has recently edited (with Marcel Verweij) a collection of original papers on public health ethics (*Ethics, prevention, and public health*, 2007, Oxford: Oxford University Press). He is joint founding editor of the new international peer-reviewed academic journal *Public Health Ethics*. For the past two years he has been Visiting Professor at the Centre for Ethics, University of Toronto, Canada.

Dr Tatiana Escobar-Koch is a medical doctor from the University of Chile. In 2008 she obtained the degree of Master of Science in Mental Health Studies with distinction from King's College London, where she won the Bouras Prize for Academic Excellence. Her research interests include bioethics and mental health. She is co-author of 'Bioethics in primary care: TB case studies' and 'Quality of informed consent documents in research with human subject protocols', both presented at the 9th World Congress of Bioethics in Croatia in 2008. She is also the first author of 'Service users' views of eating disorder services: an international comparison', published in the *International Journal of Eating Disorders* in 2009. She is currently in charge of mental health at the Cristo Vive Primary Care Family Health Centre in Santiago, Chile.

Alison Hann is a Lecturer in Public Health and Health Policy in the School of Health Science, University of Wales Swansea, UK. She undertook her doctoral research on the politics of breast cancer and continues to research and write on health policy and public health ethics with recent articles examining current screening issues. Alison is convenor of the Political Studies Association Health Politics Group. She has edited two recent texts on health policy: *Analysing Health Policy* (2000, Aldershot: Ashgate) and *Health Policy and Politics* (2007, Farnham: Ashgate).

Dr Anthony Kessel is a public health physician and medical ethicist. His current position is Director of Public Health Strategy for the UK Health Protection Agency (HPA), and Honorary Professor and Coordinator of the International Programme for Ethics, Public Health and Human Rights (IPEPH) at the London School of Hygiene & Tropical Medicine (LSHTM). Previously Anthony has been Director of Public Health at Camden Primary Care Trust in London and also a general practitioner. At the HPA Anthony is responsible for issues of national public health strategy, and oversees areas including international health, professional development, health protection governance and public health training. At the university his research interests are in public health ethics, public health policy, and environmental health. Anthony has published articles, reports and book chapters in areas such as public health ethics, clinical ethics, research ethics, HIV and environmental health He is sole author of *Air, the environment and public health* (2006, Cambridge: Cambridge University Press).

Stephen Holland is a Senior Lecturer in the Departments of Philosophy and Health Sciences at the University of York, UK. His principal research interests are in bioethics and public health ethics. Most recent work includes an article on the viability of virtue ethics as an approach to bioethics, in the journal *Bioethics*, and a piece on public health paternalism, in the journal *Public Health Ethics*. Stephen is the author of *Bioethics: A philosophical introduction* (2003, Cambridge: Polity) and *Public Health Ethics* (2007: Cambridge: Polity).

Stephen Peckham is a Reader in Health Policy in the Department of Public Health and Policy at the London School of Hygiene & Tropical Medicine. Until April 2009 he was Director of the National Coordinating Centre for the National Institutes of Health Research Service Delivery and Organisation Research Programme and remains an advisor to the programme. His main research interests are in health policy analysis and he is currently involved in research on inter-organisational aspects of performance and decentralised decision making in local health economies, patient choice, primary care and public health, and public health policy and ethics. He has published widely on health and social policy and health services research. Recent books include *Primary care in the UK* (2002, with M. Exworthy, Basingstoke: Palgrave) and *Social policy for nurses and the helping professions* (2007, with E. Meerabeau, Buckingham: Open University Press).

Marla Solari is a registered nurse. She holds a degree in social sciences from the Latin American Institute of Social Sciences (1994), a Master's degree in Bioethics from the University of Chile (1997), a diploma in Bioethics, Social Dimensions (1998), and a diploma in Research with Human Subjects Bioethics (2006). She is Director of the Cristo Vive Primary Care Family Health Centre and a member of its Bioethics Committee, and she is also a member of the Research with Human

Subjects Ethics Committee of Northern Santiago. In addition, she is Assistant Professor at the Faculty of Medicine of the University of Chile. Her research interests include bioethics, primary care public health, and ethics of research with human subjects. She is co-author of 'Bioethics in primary care: TB case studies' and 'Quality of informed consent documents in research with human subject protocols', both presented at the 9th World Congress of Bioethics in Croatia in 2008. She is also the first author of 'Attitudes and conducts of the health care team regarding the HIV/AIDS epidemic', published in the *Número Especial de Jurisprudencia Argentina sobre Derechos personalísimos, VIH/sida y prensa escrita* in 2008.

Erica Sutton is pursuing a PhD at the Dalla Lana School of Public Health and the Joint Centre for Bioethics at the University of Toronto in Ontario, Canada. Her dissertation examines the moral implications of expanded newborn screening from a critical, feminist public health ethics perspective. Erica received her Master's from McGill University in Religious Studies with a specialisation in Bioethics. She also worked for three years as a social and behavioral research fellow at the National Human Genome Research Institute at the National Institutes of Health in Bethesda, Maryland. Other research interests include public health ethics explorations of vaccination and new reproductive technologies as well as social and behavioural science research on decision-making around birth place and birth attendants, cardiac prevention and rehabilitation programmes for women, and individuals living with rare genetic conditions.

Angela Tod is a Principal Research Fellow at Sheffield Hallam University, UK. She has a clinical background in nursing but has been primarily involved in research for a number of years. Recent projects include work exploring delay in diagnosis of lung cancer, evaluation of an early warning scoring system in acute care, evaluation of a smoke-free homes initiative, public engagement in healthcare commissioning, nutrition of oncology patients in an acute setting, nurses' role and experience of breaking bad news. Angela has been a member of an NHS and university research ethics committee for over 10 years.

Dr Ross Upshur is currently the Director of the University of Toronto Joint Centre for Bioethics and Director of the Primary Care Research Unit and staff physician at the Department of Family and Community Medicine, Sunnybrook Health Sciences Centre. Dr Upshur is the Canada Research Chair in Primary Care Research. At the University of

Toronto he is a Professor in the Department of Family and Community Medicine and Dalla Lana School of Public Health, Adjunct Scientist at the Institute of Clinical Evaluative Sciences, an affiliate of the Institute of the History and Philosophy of Science and Technology and a member of the Centre for Environment. He is an Adjunct Associate Professor in the School of Geography and Earth Sciences and Associate Member of the Institute of Environment and Health at McMaster University. He is a member of The Royal College of Physicians and Surgeons of Canada and the College of Family Physicians of Canada.

ONE

Introduction: Why public health ethics?

Stephen Peckham and Alison Hann

While ethics has been a central consideration of medical research and healthcare delivery, the application of ethics to public health policy and practice is less well developed. There is, however, an increasing interest in public health ethics, reflecting a renewed international policy emphasis on public health, debates about the effectiveness of public health interventions and discussions at a global level about public health risks and action. Public health ethics is now part of mainstream public health training in the US and there is interest in developing ethical frameworks for public health policy and practice in the UK. For example, the Nuffield Council on Bioethics has recently concluded a consultation on public health ethics and published a report that has focused wider UK attention on ethical issues in public health, although the report tends to address broad issues such as obesity and infectious diseases rather than the application of ethics in public health practice. However, it does contain some guidance for local policy makers on how to approach ethical issues. In addition, concern has been expressed that the Council's approach is influenced too much by traditional bioethics and not by more recent ethical and philosophical debate about public health.

With developing technology (such as new vaccines) and new potential public health threats (for example, swine flu and resistant strains of TB), ethical issues in public health are going to be even more central than they are now. Increased mobility nationally and internationally has also changed the way countries have to think about public health issues. This also includes more ways to monitor people, the use of genetic testing, and more public awareness of threats to public health and an awareness that there are ethical and possibly legal (for example, enforced quarantine) difficulties with the distribution of harms and benefits. Balancing the rights and responsibilities of individuals and wider populations is becoming more complex. There is clearly a need to develop this debate and we hope that this book will play a key role in opening out a discussion of public health ethics into the public health practice arena, as well as provide insights into the complexities of making public health decisions in practice.

This book is the outcome of a conference held in May 2007, in Birmingham, UK, to stimulate discussion about the ethical approaches that public health practitioners adopt in practice. The conference was attended by academics from philosophical, social science and public health disciplines and by public health practitioners. Conference papers covered a wide range of public health topics and were presented by both practitioners and academics from a wide range of disciplines. Outcomes from the conference include exploring how to influence the development of ethical training for public health practitioners in the UK and other countries by working with the Faculty of Public Health and others, and raising the profile of public health ethics and the need for further research. The papers from the conference form the core of this book, which will be the first on this topic to focus on public health practice rather than on more philosophical discussions of ethics as applied to public health. The book is also very timely, given current concerns about new epidemics and public health threats.

Public health ethics

In the period since the Second World War increasing attention has been paid to ethical issues in medicine and healthcare. The focus on patient rights with respect to consent to treatment reflected a growing interest in individual rights and was a precursor of the emergence in the 1970s of biomedical ethics as a discipline, and ignited work in medical ethics, creating a distinct field of professional enquiry and establishing philosophical principles as the foundation for exploring ethical issues in medicine (Beauchamp and Childress, 1994; Gillon, 1994; R. Porter, 1999; D. Porter, 1999). Medical ethics became a central element of medical practice, and an academic discipline of medical ethics rapidly developed from the 1970s. However, in the 1990s new approaches to biomedical ethics emerged that provided a different perspective to medical ethics and challenged the central approach of medical ethics as simply the application of moral philosophy to medicine (Davis, 1995). These included care ethics (Tong, 1998), feminist and social science perspectives on medical ethics (Weisz, 1990), casuistry and historical critiques (Hoffmaster, 1994; Cooter, 1995). Medical ethics was also criticised for its narrow clinical focus, and since the late 1980s a broader conceptualisation of bioethics has emerged that sees the need for public health, environmental health and human rights to be more central to ethical discussion and health. As a result, new fields of public health ethics (Coughlin and Beauchamp, 1996; Coughlin, 1997; Calman and Downie, 1997; Darragh and McCarrick, 1998; Weed, 1999; Kessel, 2003), environmental ethics (Callicott, 1979; Des Jardins, 1997; Light and Holmes, 2003) and global bioethics (Elliot, 1993; Low, 1999) have emerged.

Today, while ethics is considered a central element of medical research and healthcare delivery, the application of ethics to public health policy and practice is less well developed (Kass, 2001; Callaghan and Jennings, 2002; Childress et al, 2002). The increasing interest in public health ethics reflects a renewed international policy emphasis on public health, debates about the effectiveness of public health interventions, discussions at a global level about public health risks and action, and the impact of policies on the health of vulnerable and disadvantaged populations (Benetar et al, 2003). Public health ethics is now part of mainstream public health training and there is interest in developing ethical frameworks for public health policy and practice (Gostin and Lazzarini, 1997; Childress et al, 2002; Kass, 2004). In the UK the Nuffield Council on Bioethics has recently concluded a consultation on public health ethics. The Council invited comments on a paper that set out key debates in public health ethics in areas such as vaccination programmes, water fluoridation, quarantine and obesity. Following a period of consultation and deliberation, the Council finally published its report in November 2007 (Nuffield Council on Bioethics, 2007).

The Nuffield Council drew on the stewardship model to define the role of governments but developed this so that "governments should not coerce people or restrict their freedom unnecessarily ... and to provide the conditions under which people can live healthy lives", but stated also that the "stewardship state" "has a particular responsibility for reducing health inequalities and protecting the health of vulnerable groups such as children" (Krebs, 2008, p 579). While it is an important contribution to raising the profile of public health ethics, the Council's report does not provide a framework for the application of ethical consideration in decision making. The Council's report is also uniquely UK focused. As many of the papers in the *Bulletin of the World Health Organization*'s special issue on public health ethics identify, public health ethics is an international topic operating within an international context (Coleman et al, 2008; McDougall et al, 2008; Petrini and Gainotti, 2008; Schrecker, 2008). This is a theme also dealt with in two chapters in this book, by Upshur on TB (Chapter Four), and by Sutton and Upshur on vaccination and public health (Chapter Eleven).

While to identify that public health decisions are rooted in ethical debates as well as in more epistemological discussions about the nature and use of evidence or the application of professional knowledge provides a useful context, it does not necessarily provide a useful aid to the practitioner or policy maker. As Kenny and Giacomini (2005) have argued, "The quintessential ethical problem of the public policy maker is how to define, identify, justify, and distribute inevitable benefits and harms, rather than simply striving to ensure benefit and avoid harm" (p 254). Public health policy, more specifically, involves not only decisions to be made about important questions relating to the degree or distribution of *health* harm or benefit, but also how to define those health harms and benefits and balance them against issues such as individual freedom. For example, a key debate in public health is the extent to which it is right to interfere with someone else's liberty in order to protect them and/or others from harm. Much of the philosophical literature and debate on public health has focused on whether public health programmes, such as childhood vaccination, maximise benefit, avoid harm or interfere with the liberty of individuals. Weed (2004) has suggested that public health is located at the crowded and difficult intersection between risk, health effects and prevention – a theme returned to throughout this book. To help practitioners and policy makers navigate their way through this contentious area there is an appeal to scientific evidence to support particular interventions and actions in public health. This appeal is primarily based within a biomedical model of health and relies on the principle that it is possible to scientifically measure benefit and harm. Such ideas link to the concept that to act ethically is to be rational – a key claim of scientific evidence.

However, it is widely recognised that evidence is not value neutral and is contestable – as seen in areas such as tobacco control or food policy – and there are a number of key methodological debates. Evidence is either philosophical–normative (independent of context), with an emphasis on the quality and criteria for evidence, or practical–operational (context-based), where evidence "is characterised by its emergent and provisional nature, being inevitably incomplete and inconclusive" (Dobrow et al, 2004, p 209). Such debates about the nature of evidence are not new. Douglas (1986) argues that the way we make sense of the world, the categories of classification, are all socially constituted and socially reproduced. Freeman (2007) has argued that public health policy making is characterised by 'bricolage', a process where the policy maker "in contrast to the scientist or engineer, acquires and assembles tools and materials as he or she goes, keeping them until they might be used". Moreover, evidence from research has to compete with "ordinary knowledge" which owes its origins to "common sense, casual empiricism or thoughtful speculation and analysis". Thus, public health policy makers, practitioners and lay people are faced with an array of evidence that supports different positions on public health action. The scientific evidence generally is seen as most definitive, even though it is sometimes ignored or overridden by other interests in the policy process. These issues are returned to in Chapter Two by Cribb, who suggests that strategies that appeal to scientific evidence or social and political authority are also forms of 'ethics avoidance'.

In public health two further issues need clarification. First, we need to be concerned with how public health problems are defined, operationalised and influenced by cultural and social norms. Second, public health ethics should also consider policy implementation, not just the outcome. Public health programmes are more likely to cause some degree of harm or restrict liberty of action, but a utilitarian approach advocates that the means are less important than the overall outcome. Yet, in public health policy and action other considerations, based on the way the outcome is achieved, are also important, and while concepts of benefit and harm are useful it is also important to consider other criteria such as truthfulness (for example about the safety of interventions), acting in good faith, openness, and so on. The development of ethical frameworks for public health will, therefore, need to consider both means and ends, and therefore utilitarian approaches are not sufficient.

It is within this complex landscape of philosophical and scientific uncertainty that public health policy is developed and practice undertaken. The Nuffield Council on Bioethics (2007) report has been an important contribution but does not address how ethical principles or concepts are applied in practice. It does, however, add to a limited literature that has attempted to develop a framework for public health ethics or to apply normative moral theory to public health (Gostin and Lazzarini, 1997; Childress et al, 2002; Kass, 2004). As Petrini and Gainotti (2008) argue, "anyone attempting to find unifying principles for public-health ethics might soon become discouraged" (p 624). Not only is it difficult to define the field of activity of public health, but the definition of public health professional is also becoming increasingly difficult (Petrini and Gainotti, 2008). In terms of application to practice, only the American Public Health Association has developed a code of ethics and placed the study of public health ethics within the professional curriculum. In contrast, the only reference to ethics within the UK public health training schemes is with reference to personal conduct. However, as argued by authors in this volume (see Holland and Upshur, for example), developing an ethical framework is not necessarily a useful starting point, as any such framework needs to be set within a practice context, framed as a statement of principles. As Petrini and Gainotti (2008) argue, this is perhaps a useful way forward, as establishing principles for action by public health professionals is something that can be identified and agreed on, and can potentially provide a basis for ethical conduct. They suggest that drawing out the key personalist concepts within such guidelines may provide such a basis. It is not the purpose here to engage with their suggestions, but rather to explore ethical issues in public health practice and policy. Thus, the purpose of the chapters in this book is to set the debate about public health ethics within a practice and policy context. To this end, we have drawn on papers presented at the Birmingham conference, together with some additional contributions. The aim is both to provide a conceptual discussion of public health ethics and also to show how ethical issues are relevant and addressed in public health practice.

This book

We have divided the book into three parts. In the first part we introduce the concept of public health ethics, and the contributions from Professor Alan Cribb and Dr Steve Holland provide two complementary approaches to thinking about how public health ethics is conceptualised and how it relates to the practice of public health. Alan Cribb's chapter provides an important opening to debates about public health ethics and how these are conceptualised. He argues that public health ethics is an integral part of public health practice and policy. Central to his argument is the need to embed public health ethics within an interdisciplinary and societal context. He emphasises the unique nature of public health ethics and places discussion and application of ethics within a discussion that draws on philosophical principles but which is not uniquely philosophical, in that public health ethics is informed by observations that social science can bring to it and the practical complexities of everyday public health practice.

In Chapter Three, Steve Holland provides a useful framework for thinking about public health ethical problems. He sees public health ethics as primarily about the relationship between government, the individual and the community and how benefit and harm are distributed between individuals and the community. He argues that rights-based approaches are limited, but for Holland public health ethics is part of medical ethics and bioethics, providing a contrasting view to that presented by Alan Cribb in the previous chapter.

The second part of the book includes chapters addressing a range of key ethical issues in public health practice and policy. They have been written by a mix of academics and practitioners and reflect a wide range of ethical issues. The aim of this part is to provide accounts of how ethical issues relate to public health policy and practice. This practice context and the dilemmas presented to public health practitioners are starkly presented by Dr Ross Upshur in his chapter on resistant tuberculosis. He directly addresses the dilemma raised by Steve Holland about the question of restraint and getting the right balance between individual rights and community protection. In this chapter Ross Upshur argues that understanding the determinants of drug-resistant tuberculosis and the emergence of the HIV/TB syndemic is crucial to applied public health ethics. The chapter summarises recent developments in tuberculosis and HIV, and applies a critical framework to analyse the failures and discuss the role of public health – including an exploration of the use of controversial measures such as isolation for the control of communicable diseases. The discussion in this chapter is clearly relevant to strategies for infectious disease containment within both national and, increasingly, international contexts.

The next chapter, by Peter Allmark, Angela Tod and Jo Abbott, raises a wider question about the value base of health promotion – an issue returned to in a later chapter on obesity. Their discussion of health promotion in relation to smoking highlights the difficulties and dilemmas of health messages even where epidemiological evidence is strong. The success of public health policy and practice is often judged by its ability to change public behaviour. The emphasis on lifestyle and the responsibility of individuals to change their behaviour has been integral to much public health policy over the years. The authors argue that insofar as health education is *education* it should be judged by the success with which it leads to people holding accurate beliefs. This would be a cognitive rather than a behavioural criterion for judging public health policies. Using examples from research on health promotion and smoking, they demonstrate that this would probably result in better outcomes. However, the cognitive criterion may sometimes be at odds with achieving optimum health outcomes, and thus the choice between them is then an important and unavoidable moral one.

Similar debates about the use of public health messages are central to the discussion of obesity in Chapter Eight, where Alison Hann and Stephen Peckham examine the nature of obesity and how it is defined in public health policy and practice.

Chapter Six provides a contrast to professionally focused approaches to public health by providing an example of how local ethical issues are dealt with in Chile. The example of the local community ethics committee within primary healthcare provides a very different model of practice from that in the UK and other western countries with a longer tradition of public health interventions and health promotion. The idea of taking ethical problems that occur in practice and debating the appropriate course of action clearly occurs in many places, but not perhaps within the more structured Primary Care Bioethics Committees. Sixty per cent of the Chilean population (including the poorest people in the country) belong to the public health system. These people are taken care of in the family primary healthcare clinics. Most of the bioethical problems which the primary care health teams have to deal with are associated with community life and social conditions. Facing these issues involves interaction between the healthcare team, the community and the health network.

The chapter by Jessica Datta and Anthony Kessel introduces another aspect of ethical debate in public health. They examine the ethical issues raised by the retention of tissue or blood for anonymous testing. Routine use of blood samples for epidemiological purposes raises a number of key ethical concerns and it is clear that other tissue has also been used for similar purposes. Recent publicity demonstrates a public concern about this issue. Such practices raise ethical issues for individuals and specific communities. They also raise ethical issues for public health and other healthcare practitioners.

Controversies about vaccinations continue to preoccupy the media, both public and scientific. It is not just high-profile debates about MMR (measles, mumps and rubella) vaccines that have found their way into the public's consciousness, but concerns over hepatitis vaccination, the human papillomavirus (HPV) vaccine and recent concern about the efficacy of flu vaccines (Jefferson, 2006) have also provided a focus for heated debate in medical circles. The last three chapters in Part Two address these debates. Chapter Nine examines the application of ethics to vaccination. In it Alison Hann and Stephen Peckham argue that justification for vaccination programmes is based on differing values and principles and that vaccination requires an exploration of ethical issues. This is followed by a chapter examining the new HPV vaccine, and Chapter Eleven by Erica Sutton and Ross Upshur discusses vaccination programmes as an approach to containing and eradicating communicable diseases.

In the first of these three chapters we discuss the ethical framework for vaccination programmes. The intention here is not to question the efficacy or otherwise of such programmes but to explore the ethical frameworks that are used to justify vaccination programmes. The chapter explores what kinds of ethical approaches public health practitioners can adopt in support of developing and implementing public health programmes. This is not without problems, and is an issue that Angus Dawson returns to in Chapter Twelve. Questions about evidence and balancing benefits and harm are central to this discussion and reflect a long-standing focus of public health ethical practice. In relation to vaccination there is a general acceptance of the benefit, with those opposing vaccination seen as irrational.

Chapter Ten examines the introduction of HPV vaccination programmes, demonstrating that public health is certainly a dynamic area of health policy and action where changing technology brings new successes and challenges for addressing public health problems. Cervical cancer is a major public health issue and many countries run screening programmes. However, cervical cancer is also the first cancer to be linked specifically with an infectious cause – HPV. There is now good evidence to demonstrate that a number of the 200 strains of HPV are implicated in cervical cancer. It is not surprising, therefore, that a substantial effort has been made to find a vaccine, and two have recently been developed by Merck and GlaxoSmithKlein. In June 2007 the UK Joint Committee on Vaccination and Immunisation recommended that the HPV vaccine should be routinely given to girls aged 12 to 13, and the countrywide programme commenced in October 2008. The mass immunisation programme against HPV presents some important ethical dilemmas for policy makers and practitioners, and the chapter examines these questions within the current context of cervical cancer prevention programmes, considering issues of efficacy and the impact of immunisation on women, and the implications for the current cervical screening programme. The chapter raises similar concerns about how public health messages are constructed and implemented in practice. In particular, it highlights the need for further consideration about the efficacy of the delivery programme and potential risks associated with this, the additional costs of delivery of such a programme, the challenge of ensuring whether continued vaccination coverage among the highest risk population, the goals of the vaccination programme and the need to continue cervical cancer screening despite a vaccination programme.

From a more international context, Erica Sutton and Ross Upshur discuss methods for containing communicable diseases. Eradicating communicable diseases worldwide has been a primary public health goal since the 19th century, and vaccination programmes comprise a significant part of that population health effort. To achieve community health, public health authorities are bestowed with policing powers whereby individual rights can be sacrificed for the greater good of the population. However, healthcare providers and scholars are encouraging public health programmes to attain their community health goals through the least coercive and intrusive means possible. Coercive strategies, once implemented by public health authorities, are discouraged today. Human rights and ethics scholars endorse public health strategies that aim to balance individual and community rights, maintaining that public health interventions that protect human rights also achieve population health. Although vaccines are considered among the most successful public health initiatives, vaccination programmes have neither escaped social injustices nor fully incorporated human rights in their approach to health. Given the recent concerns about the swine flu pandemic and calls for measures such as mandatory vaccination, coupled with the 2007 decision by the State of Michigan to render the HPV vaccine compulsory, questions of human rights and social justice become increasingly important. This chapter discusses key aspects of the vaccination debate and shows how critical, philosophical examination of vaccination discourse, informed through a public health ethics framework that incorporates human rights, can contribute positively to future discussions and policy decisions surrounding vaccination programmes.

The third part of the book attempts to bring theory and practice together and raise key questions for future debate and discussion. Angus Dawson's chapter returns to the broader topic of theory and practice. He examines what contribution the various chapters of the book make to our understanding of public health ethics, and also how lessons from these case studies could help the development of a coherent approach to public health ethics. The chapter opens by asserting that public health ethics provides an arena of discussion missing from traditional medical ethics, and challenges the view that there are theorists and practitioners who constitute two unified and separate camps. As Dawson rightly points out, there is often little unity about what constitutes ethical practice or how public health ethics is theorised. What Dawson offers in this chapter is a way through what he describes as a continent of confusion and muddle. In essence, it is an argument for, and defence of, the role of the state in public health. While such an approach has clear advantages, it also rests on key assumptions that are tackled in the book. For example, Dawson refers to arguments in a number of chapters in this book (Hann and Peckham, Datta and Kessel, Allmark et al) about the balance of individual liberty (or rights) and the right of the state to intervene or act. Yet central to this debate is the question of the strength of evidence. Clearly, the justification for state action or resistance to interventions is often rooted in the availability and interpretation of evidence. While frameworks for public health ethics may help us to examine public health action, certainty about the evidence underpinning decisions needs to be examined as well, as much 'public health evidence', as demonstrated in the chapters in this book, is open to challenge and debate.

The final chapter draws together the various arguments in the book and reflects on what further work needs to be done to develop public health ethics. The book concludes by acknowledging the importance of ethical decision making for public health ethics. The chapter returns to the government, individual and community framework set out by Steve Holland in Chapter Three and explores the roles of government and of practitioners. These roles are explored in a number of chapters in relation to the need to balance individual and community benefit/ harm. The chapter also sets a discussion of ethics within the broader discussion of public health problems and solutions, showing how the roles of government and practitioners need to draw more clearly on ethical analysis to provide clearer guidance for public health practice. Finally, Peckham and Hann discuss how such an approach can be taken forward through research and education to support professional practice. What kinds of training and education are appropriate for public health practitioners and how should this be developed in practice? Currently, the Faculty of Public Health in the UK does not have any substantive ethical component to its public health training scheme and ethics is not one of the key competencies for public health practitioners. This is not unusual, as only the American Public Health Association has incorporated ethics within its professional guidelines and code of conduct, and ethics is also more widely taught as part of public health training in the US.

References

Beauchamp, T. and Childress, J. (1994) *Principles of biomedical ethics*, New York: Oxford University Press.

Benetar, S.R., Daar, A.S. and Singer, P. (2003) 'Global health ethics: the rationale for mutual caring', *International Affairs*, vol 79, no 1, pp 107–38.

Callaghan, D. and Jennings, B. (2002) 'Ethics and public health: forging a strong relationship', *American Journal of Public Health*, vol 92, no 2, pp 169-76.

Callicott, J.B. (1979) 'Elements of an environmental ethic: moral considerability and the biotic community', *Environmental Ethics*, vol 1, pp 71–81.

Calman, K.C. and Downie, R.S. (1997) 'Ethical principles and ethical issues in public health', in R. Detels, W.W. Holland, J. McEwen and G.S. Omenn (eds) *Oxford textbook of public health, volume 1: The scope of public health* (3rd edn), Oxford: Oxford University Press, 1997, pp 391–402.

Childress, J.F., Faden, R.R., Gaare, R.D. et al (2002) 'Public health ethics: mapping the terrain', *Journal of Law, Medicine and Ethics*, vol 30, pp 170–8.

Coleman, C.H., Bouësseau, M.C. and Reis, A. (2008) 'The contribution of ethics to public health', *Bulletin of the World Health Organization*, vol 86, pp 578–9.

Cooter, R. (1995) 'The resistible rise of medical ethics', *Society for the History of Medicine*, vol 8, no 2, pp 257–70.

Coughlin, S.S. (1997) *Ethics in epidemiology and public health practice*, Columbus, OH: Quill.

Coughlin, S.S. and Beauchamp, T.L. (eds) (1996) *Ethics and epidemiology*, New York: Oxford University Press.

Darragh, M. and McCarrick, P.M. (1998) 'Public health ethics: health by the numbers', *Kennedy Institute of Ethics Journal*, vol 8, no 3, pp 339–58.

Davis, R. (1995) 'The principlism debate: a critical overview', *Journal of Medical Philosophy*, vol 20, pp 85–105.

Des Jardins, J.R. (1997) *Environmental ethics: An introduction to environmental philosophy*. Belmont: Wadsworth.

Dobrow, M.I., Goel, V. and Upshur, R.E. (2004) 'Evidence-based health policy: context and utilisation', *Social Science and Medicine*, vol 58, pp 207-17.

Douglas, M. (1986) *How institutions think*, Syracuse, NY: Syracuse University Press.

Elliot, R. (1993) 'Environmental ethics', in P. Singer (ed) *A companion to ethics*, Oxford: Blackwell, pp 284–93.

Freeman, R. (2007) 'Epistemological bricolage: how practitioners make sense of learning', *Administration and Society*, vol 39, no 4, pp 476–96.

Gillon, R. (1994) 'Medical ethics: four principles and attention to scope', *British Medical Journal*, vol 309, pp 184–8.

Gostin, L.O. and Lazzarini, Z. (1997) *Human rights and public health in the AIDS pandemic*, New York: Oxford University Press.

Hoffmaster, B. (1994) 'The forms and limits of medical ethics', *Social Science and Medicine*, vol 39, no 9, pp 1155–64.

Jefferson, T. (2006) 'Influenza vaccination: policy versus evidence', *British Medical Journal*, no 333, pp 912-15.

Kass, N.E. (2001) 'An ethics framework for public health', *Public Health Matters*, vol 91, no 11, pp 1776–82.

Kass, N.E. (2004) 'Public health ethics: from foundations and frameworks to justice and global public health', *Journal of Law, Medicine and Ethics*, vol 32, pp 232–42.

Kenny, N. and Giacomini, M. (2005) 'Wanted: a new ethics field for health policy analysis', *Health Care Analysis*, vol 13, no 4, pp 247–60.

Kessel, A.S. (2003) 'Public health ethics education in the United Kingdom: questionnaire survey', *Social Science*, vol 56, pp 1439–45.

Krebs, J. (2008) 'The importance of public health ethics', *Bulletin of the World Health Organization*, vol 86, no 8, p 579.

Light, A. and Holmes, R. III (eds) (2003) *Environmental ethics: An anthology*, Oxford: Blackwell.

Low, N. (ed) (1999) *Global ethics and environment*, London: Routledge.

McDougall, C.W., Upshur, R.E.G. and Wilson, K. (2008) 'Emerging norms for the control of emerging epidemics', *Bulletin of the World Health Organization*, vol 86, pp 643–5.

Nuffield Council on Bioethics (2007) *Public health: Ethical issues*, London: Nuffield Council on Bioethics.

Petrini, C. and Gainotti, S. (2008) 'A personalist approach to public-health ethics', *Bulletin of the World Health Organization*, vol 86, pp 624–9.

Porter, D. (1999) *Health, civilization and the state: A history of public health from ancient to modern times*, London: Routledge.

Porter, R. (1999) *The greatest benefit to mankind: A medical history of humanity from antiquity to the present*, London: Fontana.

Schrecker, T. (2008) 'Denaturalizing scarcity: a strategy of enquiry for public-health ethics', *Bulletin of the World Health Organization*, vol 86, pp 600–5.

Tong, R. (1998) 'The ethics of care: a feminist virtue ethics of care for healthcare practitioners', *Journal of Medical Philosophy*, vol 23, no 2, pp 131–53.

Weed, D.L. (1999) 'Towards a philosophy of public health', *Journal of Epidemiology and Community Health*, vol 53, pp 99–104.

Weed, D.L. (2004) 'Precaution, prevention and public health ethics', *Journal of Medical Philosophy'*, vol 29, pp 313–32.

Weisz, G. (ed) (1990) *Social science perspectives on medical ethics*, Dordrecht: Kluwer Academic Publishers.

Part One
Public health: contexts

TWO

Why ethics? What kind of ethics for public health?

Alan Cribb

It would be very odd to insist that clinical health professionals should be mindful of, and conscientious about, the ethical issues raised in their one-to-one clinical encounters without setting similar expectations for those who work with whole populations. But – as I will suggest (and indeed this book shows more generally) – public health ethics raises many deep-seated and testing philosophical and practical challenges and those who work in, and are concerned with, public health have plenty of important things to be getting on with, without getting bogged down in an academic ethics seminar. So can we develop the field of public health ethics in a way that does justice to the imperatives of ethics and the imperatives of public health? Can we have an ethics *for* public health? With these questions in mind I will use this chapter to briefly review some of the philosophical, methodological, professional and policy challenges raised by the project of public health ethics.

Ethics avoidance

One way to deal with the many challenges inherent in public health ethics is to engage in what I will call – just to be slightly provocative – 'ethics avoidance'. This is a widespread phenomenon both inside and outside public health contexts. Ethics avoidance encompasses a range of potential strategies. Here I will just mention three popular strategies which can be combined in various ways. First, there is 'technicism' – this means treating all issues as if they were fully susceptible to technical reasoning and practical problem-solving techniques. For example, given that we are committed to reducing population levels of morbidity and mortality (and/or some other end) then we must focus on identifying and implementing the best evidence-based methods of achieving this (or other) end. This latter can then be treated essentially as a scientific-technical question which we can – and arguably should – address without being distracted by ethical speculations. Second, there is an approach that might be called 'conformism' or 'compliance' and rests on an appeal to social and political authority. This approach consists in saying "It is not up to me to decide what ought to be done. Other people (managers, official agencies, the government) are properly charged with that kind of responsibility. My role is to do my job properly." In practice this might, for instance, entail accepting the framework of targets that has been adopted by a local authority under a nationally defined programme and working with a technical and problem-solving mindset to deliver on those targets. Third, there is an appeal to 'public opinion' or some generalised notion of a democratic mandate – for example, by 'testing' the acceptability of proposed interventions through a process of consultation with potentially affected parties (to coin an ugly word, we might, therefore, call this 'acceptabilism'). Obtaining a sufficient degree of support or popular authorisation can thus be treated as a substitute for, or perhaps as a form of, ethical validation. Clearly, strategies two and three are easily combined in those instances where we envisage the source of authority (perhaps the government) as possessing a measure of democratic authorisation.

Strategies of ethics avoidance flourish because they allow us to steer clear of the deep-seated puzzles generated by thinking about ethics and they allow us to get on with confronting practical public health problems. A world in which we each had to believe we had resolved all relevant ethical dilemmas before we could 'go to work' is not necessarily a desirable world to live in – far from it. Having said that, I would also contend that ethics avoidance simply won't do. Each of the three strategies I have mentioned has a place – indeed each can be said to have some ethical relevance (that is, 'what works' matters; there is a place for authority, and 'democracy' or some notion akin to 'consent' is ethically significant). But a few minutes' reflection should indicate why, taken individually or together, these strategies are not an adequate basis for ethically defensible policy making. We know from many other circumstances that popular support (or some simple conception of democratic approval) is not a litmus test for what is right or good – all kinds of atrocities can be 'authorised' in this manner. The same applies to appeals to social or political authority – the claim that "I am only doing my job" is notorious for being an inadequate response to ethical challenges. Finally, technicism fails on two counts. It leaves aside the central question of what we ought to do, and it treats policy or practice decision making as if it were simply about finding the most effective means to specified ends, when means and ends are not so easily separated out and when there is much at stake in deciding how we should act and not just in deciding what we ought to be aiming at.

Ethical debates are intrinsic to public health. Furthermore, ethical issues are frequently recognised and deliberated about in public health policy and practice (even if not always explicitly using the language of 'ethics'). It is, for example, common to have discussions about whether certain policies take proper account of, and are respectful towards, differences in the preferences, identities and cultures of individuals and groups. It is equally commonplace to hear concerns about fairness or social justice – asking, for example, whether the benefits and burdens of public health initiatives fall in the right places. These are some of the key ways in which the 'rights and wrongs' of public health are routinely discussed. Debates about the potential and actual 'harms and benefits' produced by public health work are even more widespread. Indeed this concern with identifying the 'goods' produced or undermined by interventions is at the heart of the scientific-technical approach to public health. These preoccupations (with respect, with fairness, with harms and with benefits) reflect the core business of ethics and are famously summarised in the oft-cited 'four principles' of healthcare ethics (Beauchamp and Childress, 2001).

The disciplinary and professional cultures of public health thus provide both good news and bad news for anyone wishing to strengthen the field of public health ethics. There is widespread recognition of the ethical dimensions of public health decision making but there is, I would suggest, also a tendency not to focus sustained and systematic attention on these issues, and sometimes to positively avoid them either by conflating ethical questions with technical questions or by 'assigning them' to someone else. Ethical issues have a philosophical component, that is to say they concern questions which cannot be satisfactorily addressed by purely empirical or logical means. Rather, they require a capacity to engage in open-ended deliberation and argument about rival and often equally plausible (or apparently compelling) positions. What is needed from public health practitioners, I will suggest, is not necessarily an enthusiasm for, or expertise in, this kind of philosophical reasoning (some may well have these qualities, but it is not reasonable to expect them from everyone, just as it is not reasonable to expect interest or expertise in statistics from everyone), but simply an acknowledgement of this philosophical dimension, and a willingness, in dialogue with others, to take it seriously. I will also suggest, however, that philosophy is by no means enough. Public health ethics – if it is to be useful as well as rigorous – also depends on academic interdisciplinarity and on immersion in the contexts of practice.

The nature (and relative distinctiveness) of public health ethics

Discussions about public health ethics often begin by emphasising its distinctiveness. I will follow this precedent. In particular, in the remainder of this chapter I will focus on the kinds of questions and the kinds of methods that, I suggest, mark out public health ethics as rather different from clinical ethics. However, I should also stress that in reinforcing this notion of distinctiveness I am also quite deliberately overstating some of the differences between public health ethics and clinical ethics. This is in part because there is considerable practical overlap between the concerns of clinical healthcare and those of public health; but also – and I have tried to argue this at greater length elsewhere (Cribb, 2005) – because the ethical issues that arise at population levels are also, in various respects, relevant to clinical ethics, that is, clinical ethics ought itself to be understood in the context of public health ethics.

One way of approaching the relative distinctiveness of public health is to see that public health cuts across the boundaries of the professional and the political realms. In some respects traditional constructions of professionalism and the professional–client relationship can be applied to public health, but in other ways they break down or at least have to be rethought. On the one hand, public health work can be treated as a form of professional work, as something done by specific sets of practitioners and as thereby subject, for example, to theories about professionalism and professional virtues. On the other hand, analysing public health means taking an interest in much broader and more diffuse public policy processes and, for example, in competing political ideologies. This ambiguity about the relevance of the professional–client model applies to the population orientation of public health (that is, who is the client?); to the teamworking and intersectoral dimensions of public health work (that is, who is the professional?); and to the future and preventive orientations of public health – that is, if there is a client, they are not necessarily asking for help or being 'treated' in relation to current needs. This means that when we ask key questions in public health ethics we do so from a position which can feel unbounded by and somehow adrift from the familiar conventions of healthcare professional ethics. Specifically, problems of agency and responsibility are always to the fore in public health ethics – it is always relevant to ask "*who* has responsibility for what?". One of the things at stake is the 'division of ethical labour' – the question of the respective responsibilities of the government, other institutional agencies, individual citizens and health professionals, including public health practitioners.

Public health ethics – two key questions

There are various ways in which the core questions of public health ethics could be stated and classified. Here I will just provide a summary account of two broad indicative questions which will, I hope, also serve to further illustrate the distinctiveness of the domain. I will review them in a very general and abstract way, but it may be worth underlining the fact that they will not arise in this general form but will be embedded in specific substantive questions about what to do in relation to diverse public health agendas.

What are the goals of public health?

This question can be unpacked into a range of smaller questions. There are, for example, questions about the conceptions of health employed in public health – how far ought we to be focusing upon narrow but clinically well-defined conceptions of morbidity, or using broader and more diffuse notions such as well-being or quality of life? This is a complicated but very familiar conundrum and I won't dwell on it here except to stress that this is not just a dispute about indicators or measures, but is a dispute about what – ultimately – matters (or at least what ought to be the proper business of public health).

Public health also gives rise to overlapping and analogous questions about the conceptions of 'public' in public health – that is, there are both informal and technically defined conceptions of 'public goods' as opposed to individual goods. Many public health initiatives are aimed at ends that are provided and experienced collectively. For example, a community development team may help support work on green spaces or cycle ways both as means of promoting healthy life-styles and for the intrinsic benefits they bring. These are very different 'goods' from the exercise bike or the over-the-counter medicines that individuals may buy and use for themselves precisely because they contribute something to the community way of life – they are shared goods or common goods, and they embody and support forms of relatedness and not just individual outcomes. In the technical sense (derived from economic analysis but also deployed in the philosophical literature), public goods have the properties of being 'indivisible' (not separable out into separate units), 'non-excludable' (open to being enjoyed by all and not confined to private hands) and 'cooperation dependent' (owing their existence to the cooperation of many) (Klosko, 1987; Dawson and Verweij, 2007). Many of the goods that public health is concerned with – such as 'clean' air or herd immunity – are public goods in this sense. But we can use the idea of public goods in an extended and less formal sense simply to mean 'collective goods' and to underline the distinctive orientation of public health towards groups and communities as something over and above a collection of individuals. For example, access to clinical health services can be treated as an individual good. But the idea of a community underpinning individual access to healthcare represents something more than an aggregation of individual goods – it can be seen to embody forms of relational or civic goods such as 'solidarity'. The tensions between population-oriented goods (whether or not 'public goods' in the technical sense) and individual goods come to a head when something that is deemed beneficial for a population causes harms of one kind or another to specific individuals (I will discuss this further in relation to the next question).

Finally, the focus upon collective goods raises related but distinctive concerns about health inequalities. How far, and in what respects, is it the function of public health to address health inequalities? In some ways a focus on using public health efforts effectively will coincide with a concern with addressing inequalities in health – because, up to a point, resources directed towards the less-advantaged have the potential to enhance 'health outcomes' (however defined) most effectively. But in many cases there is an apparent tension between these two sets of concerns – for example, sometimes resources directed at 'hard to reach' groups may yield very few public health benefits as compared with resources invested in better-off populations. Here we are faced with very difficult technical and ethical choices, including choices between effectiveness and efficiency on the one hand, and equity and solidarity on the other. (And, of course, for anyone who accepts an analysis like Richard Wilkinson's (2006), that equity and solidarity may themselves be causally implicated in the production of overall health and well-being outcomes, this balancing act is reframed and further complicated.) I will not say much more about health inequalities here, but will return to this theme in the conclusion.

In short, public health faces continuous contests about narrow versus broad conceptions of health, about public versus individual goods, and about efficiency versus equality. These diverse concerns about the ends of public health can be used to illustrate the peculiar complexity of public health ethics. I can underline this point by drawing a crude – indeed exaggerated – contrast with clinical ethics. If we imagine a patient in need of a hip replacement consulting a doctor, we can envisage a whole range of possible ethical issues arising. For example, where on the waiting list should the patient be placed, in how much detail should the doctor outline the possible complications of the operation to the patient, and so on? However, the ethical issues in this instance seem largely to relate to the 'when' and the 'how' of treatment rather than to the 'what'; that is, in the specified scenario there is a mutual understanding of and agreement about the core goals. When it comes to public health, things are very rarely like this. There is almost always a great deal of contestability about goals, about *what* we should be collectively aiming at, and (as I just noted above) about *who* should be responsible for decisions and actions. Public health ethics is inherently multi-dimensional and, in particular, ethical issues about means or methods always occur alongside, and are entangled with, ethical issues about ends.

How ought we to balance population health promotion with the interests and freedoms of individuals?

This question (or some formulation of a similar question) is arguably the most prominent ethical question facing proposed public health interventions. It is one aspect of the broader tension between collective and individual ends mentioned above. By their very nature, public health interventions require the 'orchestration' of, or some degree of 'interference' in, social life and social practices. This raises obvious concerns about individual liberty. Some interventions are directly and straightforwardly coercive, including the enforcement of quarantine for highly contagious and dangerous diseases or legally enforced restrictions on life-style choices. Others involve the use of incentives or disincentives (such as using taxes or welfare subsidies to penalise or reward certain individual choices). Some are non-coercive, but even these may still raise legitimate concerns about the possibility of some degree of compromise to individual autonomy (such as social marketing messages that socially valorise or condemn certain practices). This is a huge topic in itself which – like all ethics – merits analysis on a case-by-case basis. To most people it will seem comparatively easy to rule out extreme positions – one that places no value on individual liberty when set against population health outcomes, or one that warrants no compromise to liberty, no matter how great the risks or benefits. But there is a large range of possible intermediate positions and there is no non-contentious way of arbitrating between them. This is an area where the political nature of public health is evident. The rival demands of, and potential balancing of, more liberal and more communitarian conceptions of the good society is a long-standing debate within political philosophy. Even in terms of crude party politics, the frequent mud-slinging around the spectre of the 'nanny state' provides a pragmatic political consideration which requires public health workers to tread carefully in policy making.

At the risk of, yet again, over-simplifying the distinction between clinical ethics and public health ethics, it could be said that the default position of clinical ethics (at least according to contemporary western bioethics) centres on respect for the individual patient and his or her autonomy, whereas the default position of public health ethics centres on the pursuit of the collective or common good. By its very nature, public health aims first and foremost at promoting population benefit and thus has a broadly 'utilitarian' orientation, that is, it tends to place an emphasis on maximising overall 'output' rather than to focus upon 'gains and losses' at the level of the individual. Of course it does not follow from the fact that public health *tends* to be like this that it *ought* to be – but, on the other hand, there are arguably limits to how far it is practicable to have public health as a deliberate aim and at the same time to be highly sensitive and responsive to every possible instance where some individual interest is or seems to be compromised. Nonetheless, the competing ethical demands of treating individual people (and groups) with respect and with fairness do generate a constant stream of ethical dilemmas for public health policy and practice and provide a critical check on the concern with population utility.

It is important to stress that the two broad questions reviewed above are only illustrative. For example, the ethical tension between population health and individual liberty, although important, is only one such tension. There are other population ends (apart from health) which are relevant to public health work – as I indicated above, for example, a concern with solidarity and/or equality can perfectly properly be part of the business of public health, and pursuing these ends may also conflict with the interests and freedoms of individuals. Similarly, there are, in addition to autonomy, a range of other 'individual goods' at stake – such as questions of privacy or confidentiality raised by forms of surveillance and population data collection. Also it is important to distinguish between utilitarian and paternalistic reasons for health promotion; that is, to distinguish between the tensions between 'your health' and 'my autonomy' on the one hand (for example, restricting my ability to practise shooting in public spaces) and between 'my health' and 'my autonomy' on the other (for example, restricting my ability to consume great quantities of sugar). In the latter case the question that arises is when, if ever, it can be justifiable for someone to override my autonomy with the express intention of promoting my health and welfare. This is a question about the justifiability of public health paternalism. Because 'paternalism' is often used, in popular discourse, as a straightforwardly pejorative expression, it is worth stressing that paternalism is not regarded as an inherently 'bad' thing in ethics. Rather, there is an open debate as to when, where and why paternalism may be justifiable.

In addition to technicism and the other strategies of 'ethics avoidance', I have now mentioned three of the 'occupational risks' facing an ethics of public health practice: 'healthism' (taking health as an overriding value), unqualified utilitarianism (taking population utility as an overriding value) and 'paternalism' (overriding the wishes of individuals 'for their own good'). Each of these tendencies may well have a place in an ethically defensible public health policy, but each requires justification, some degree of qualification and balancing with other relevant values.

Public health ethics – what methods are needed?

As I have hinted, I take it for granted that public health ethics will draw upon moral and political philosophy. These are the disciplines that have specific expertise in relation to contests about the nature of, and justification of, ethical and political judgements. To stress the central importance of moral and political philosophy is not just to engage in an exercise of 'professional closure' (that is, "We own this domain, so keep out of it unless you are one of us") – there are very good epistemological and practical reasons to turn to philosophy in this arena. Philosophy has produced: (1) very strong practices of argumentative rigour in relation to ethics, which means that claims and counter claims are subjected to continuous intellectual 'audit'; (2) a tradition of developing and debating rich and competing sets of theoretical resources (such as around varieties of consequentialism, or rights theory or communitarianism etc) through which ethical positions can be articulated, compared, critiqued and defended; and (3) a very diverse and substantial body of literature which analyses substantive ethical issues in depth and detail (including work on public health-related themes). For all of these reasons I would claim that philosophical methods must have a central place in the methodology of public health ethics.

Philosophy is especially important here, I would argue, to combat some of the technicist tendencies in public health cultures mentioned above. It is very easy for technicist currents to 'colonise' public health ethics, because many of the key issues in public health ethics can be usefully presented in a form that is analogous to technical decision making. Specifically, public health ethics can be presented as either (1) a form of cost–benefit analysis in which the global ethical 'costs' and 'benefits' of alternatives have to be weighed together, and/or (2) a kind of decision making by formula in which a decision tree is followed (for example: Are the population health benefits high? Is the restriction of individual liberty low? Has the rationale been publicly spelled out? Has some (practicable) provision been made for minorities who object? etc). These are in some ways useful (and broadly sensible) ways of thinking about ethics; however, the surface resemblances to, and apparent analogies with, technical decision making are misleading because ethical reasoning cannot be completely translated into these technical models – what is at issue is inherently qualitative and not purely quantitative, each of the values in question is open to multiple competing interpretations, and their relative importance is fundamentally contestable (as is the nature of any decision process, including forms of 'weighing' costs and benefits). In short, ethics requires some philosophy.[1]

Any further specification of methods will depend upon what we think public health ethics is for. If we see public health ethics as a branch of academic ethics concerned with broad questions of principle (of the sort illustrated above) then philosophical methods will be sufficient. However, if we see public health ethics as having a practical function – and in particular, as directly relevant to policy makers and practitioners in public health – then philosophy is not enough. Public health ethics needs to be both academically interdisciplinary and also 'closer to the ground'. A practice-oriented public health ethics must draw heavily on empirical research and a range of social science scholarship. I am using 'social sciences' here in a very broad sense to refer to all that scholarly work that aims to produce a systematic (and self-critical) account of the nature of the social world. Other aspects of the study of public health place great emphasis upon scientific rigour and on making evidence-based judgements (albeit that there are legitimate debates about reductionist tendencies within the specific ideology of the evidence-based movement itself). There are overwhelmingly strong reasons for this – the potential for harms or benefits being produced in the name of public health are immense, and for that reason we need to have as much confidence as possible in the empirical judgements deployed in public health practice. Exactly the same applies in public health ethics. Judgements about what ought to be done depend upon careful judgements about the causes and effects of health-related phenomena and about the possible consequences of the interventions under consideration.

But this way of putting things does not really bring out what I see as either the nature of, or the importance of, interdisciplinarity. It creates the impression that social sciences (along with clinical sciences) should simply be regarded as a resource for healthcare ethics – that they provide accounts of 'the facts' which add to the toolkit of ethics, but that they do not make a direct or significant contribution to thinking about ethical issues in public health. My own view is that this is mistaken. Public health ethics is highly context sensitive, and the social sciences make a crucial contribution to understanding contexts – providing not simply an account of 'facts' but also analytical and theoretical readings of empirical reality and, in plain terms, a 'feel' for the social world. In calling public health ethics context sensitive, I simply mean that the ethical judgements we make will depend upon culture and history and will be – at least to some extent – path dependent; that is, what it is possible to do or achieve depends upon the structures and cultures already in existence, the policy battles that have already been won and lost, and what platforms have thereby been built for further action. Both political philosophy and practical political judgement are therefore relevant to making public health judgements.

In highlighting this I am not signing up to any kind of epistemological relativism. I am just acknowledging something much more mundane – namely, that ethical issues often rest upon very difficult balancing acts which are rarely decisively resolved and that even small differences from case to case can make all the difference. There are complex questions about the relationship between philosophical ethics and empirical ethics which I will not attempt to address here, but my own starting point is that ethical reasoning is not simply applied *to* cases but is done *through* cases. What I am calling context, in other words, is not just a backcloth but is something constitutive of actions and outcomes – so what is at stake is *different* from one instance to another and from one set of circumstances to another. To take just one example: striking the ethically most defensible balance between imposing restrictions on and strengthening education about alcohol usage (or other life-style factors) will depend to some degree on time and place, because what these things mean, and therefore amount to, will vary across time and place.

But the fact that public health issues are socially and culturally constituted is not the only reason that context sensitivity is of critical importance. Attention to contexts matters because public health is about the whole social stage and not just particular scenarios or actions. This means, for example, that specific interventions need to be evaluated as part of an overall pattern of provision and expectation – thus, for instance, if we want to know whether or not it is reasonable for a government to make certain demands on people in pursuit of a particular public health goal, it is important to think about the whole 'package' of expectations and entitlements to which they are subject, including what level of government support and other resources they enjoy 'in return' (see, for example, Erin and Harris (1993) on reciprocity). In addition – and I do not think this point can be over-stressed – any consideration of the social stage and of packages of services and demands needs to be based on people's experiences on the ground and not on official policy plans or declarations. This requires a combination of close empirical work and practical immersion in the field.

And there is a further, more theoretical, contribution that social sciences can make to public health ethics which arises from the critical currents within the social sciences. In healthcare ethics there is sometimes a tendency for ethicists to take problems up in the terms that they are presented by policy makers and practitioners. Critical social scientists (and some philosophers) exhibit the opposite tendency, that is, to problematise or deconstruct the official framing of problems. This has huge implications for public health ethics. If we take the official framing of certain 'public health problems' as our starting point, then we will have started doing our ethics too far 'downstream'. The broad point – which I have elaborated further elsewhere (Cribb, 2007) – is that the categories and frameworks of public health have value judgements embedded in them and these feed into policies and practices that have effects; for example, the ways in which public health problems and solutions are constructed may reinforce certain moralising discourses, may alter the distribution of health experiences whether narrowly or broadly conceived, or may produce or reproduce patterns of discrimination or stigmatisation. Critical social science provides powerful tools to help expose and illuminate these dangers and, for this reason, enriches ethical reasoning.

But of course the main difference between an academic ethicist (however interdisciplinary) and a practitioner is not just that the latter has to think carefully about the issue in relation to particular contexts, but that they have to *do* something or other. The resources of applied philosophy and the social sciences have to be put to the service of practical judgement and, indeed, of practical politics. That is, in a practical public health ethics we do need to give some thought to what could be achieved and publicly defended within particular communities. I say 'could be', not 'can be', because I do not want to exclude the possibility that transformations might be achievable in the ways people think and act – otherwise I would be guilty of advocating simple 'acceptabilism'. However, I am equally wary of advocating any species of inert idealism – in which what ought to be done is demonstrated, with rigour, to a world that is simply not listening to what it sees as a disconnected voice. The real challenge is to do 'applied ethics', and, I am suggesting, the job of 'application' is part of ethics, not complementary to it; that is, it seems to me that ethics is not done and then applied, but is done, at least in part, in its application.

Conclusion

To conclude, I will start another discussion. I want to very briefly open up the question of health inequalities – a subject which is immensely complex empirically and theoretically, and very thorny from an ethical and political perspective. Nonetheless, it is a suitable subject through which to illustrate and summarise the themes of this chapter.

Many in the public health community believe that health inequalities are of substantial importance both epidemiologically and ethically (although the reasons for, meanings of, and implications of this belief are subject to considerable debate). For the purposes of this discussion I will assume that they are right in this belief. Given this premise, it is comparatively easy to see why a narrow approach to public health ethics will not do. If we are asked to consider the 'ethics' of a particular intervention (for example, a new screening modality), then it makes sense to examine the particular properties of the intervention, that is, how effective is it, whether appropriate education is provided, whether some people are excluded from benefiting from the intervention, and so on. This is an important part of public health ethics. However, in addressing these questions, other larger and more 'external' questions will, or at least should, arise. For example: Why is this particular disease category being used and targeted? Is our public health strategy too medicalised? How does the proposed intervention affect the overall burden of health and illness in society? These broader questions are also an important part of public health ethics.

It should be clear that a full consideration of the relevant ethical issues means addressing the broader 'external' questions and not simply the narrower questions about the properties of the intervention, and also that addressing the broader questions involves the consideration of even broader philosophical questions about the purposes of public health, the nature of the good society and the role of public health in pursuing or underpinning the good society. So if, as we are assuming, we think that health inequalities are of considerable ethical importance, we cannot merely treat them as one consideration among many which can be kept off the agenda and on the shelf while tackling more routine and technical-seeming ethical evaluations of specific interventions. (Or, to be more precise, we cannot simply assume that this is possible.) Rather, we need to be ready to practise public health ethics with philosophical questions (for example, about the meaning and importance of health equality) centre stage.

But, as I have also suggested, it would be a mistake to imagine that tackling these philosophical questions is enough. Even if we can imagine demonstrating, to the satisfaction of both philosophy and public health colleagues, that public health policy ought to be substantially reconfigured around the goal of more equal 'health opportunities' (again, something that seems to me and many others to be broadly right), then the work of ethics here has only just begun. Unless the public health community mounts a political coup and takes on very extensive policing powers itself (which in any case would require a great deal of ethical justification!), then much thought and effort will need to go into determining what – in practical terms – can justifiably be done, by whom, to further this project. There are, of course, many things that public health practitioners could do themselves in this connection. There is a long and much-celebrated tradition of advocacy in public health, and a closely associated and equally important tradition of public education. As more and more people come to understand that equal access to health depends on so much more than equal access to health services, then the climate of practical politics changes. Advocacy and education about these matters has, in my opinion, been one of the major contributions of the public health tradition. Public health ethics needs to proceed as much through these step-by-step practical developments as through overarching philosophical argument.

Note
[1] To be clear, I am suggesting that technicism poses a double threat to ethics – it can keep ethics off the agenda or it can 'take it over' once it is on the agenda.

References

Beauchamp, T.L. and Childress, J.F. (2001) *Principles of biomedical ethics*, Oxford: Oxford University Press.

Cribb, A. (2005) *Health and the good society*, Oxford: Oxford University Press.

Cribb, A. (2007) 'Health promotion, society and health care ethics', in R. Ashcroft, A. Dawson, H. Draper and J. McMillan (eds) *Principles of health care ethics*, Chichester: John Wiley and Sons.

Dawson, A. and Verweij, M. (2007) *Ethics, prevention and public health*, Oxford: Oxford University Press.

Erin, C. and Harris, J. (1993) 'AIDS: ethics, justice and social policy', *Journal of Applied Philosophy*, vol 10, no 2, pp 165–73.

Klosko, G. (1987) 'Presumptive benefit, fairness and political obligation', *Philosophy and Public Affairs*, vol 16, no 3, pp 241–59.

Wilkinson, R. (2006) *The impact of inequality: How to make sick societies healthier*, London: Routledge.

THREE

Public health ethics: what it is and how to do it

Stephen Holland

This chapter is in two parts. The first asks what public health ethics is, and defends a conception of the subject. The second asks how we should go about doing public health ethics, and presents two lines of thought about methodologies.

What is public health ethics?

The central problematic

Public health ethics centres on a problematic triad. The members of the triad are governments, populations and individuals. The triad is problematic because populations and individuals sometimes clash: the rights and freedoms of individuals can come into tension with the need to protect and promote the health of the population. In such circumstances, the government has the role of adjudicating between the two claimants. Sometimes the government sides with individuals and protects their rights and freedoms at the expense of communal health benefits. Sometimes the government sides with a community by protecting and promoting its health at the expense of individual rights and freedoms. But whichever way it is resolved, this problematic triad is central to public health ethics (Holland, 2007, pp viii–ix).

To illustrate, smoking undermines the public's health by making smokers ill and threatening the health of bystanders. So there is a clash between the individual's freedom to choose to smoke and the need to protect the community from the detrimental effects of smoking. With which of these two claimants does the government side? Focusing on the UK, legislation was passed in 2007 banning smoking in certain public places. Evidently, this represents a shift towards prioritising the need to protect the health of the population over individuals' rights to choose to smoke wherever they like. But note that this is no more than a shift in priorities, because the official rationale for the ban is that it will protect bystanders such as bar staff and restaurant workers from the effects of secondary smoking, hence it does not outlaw smoking altogether but allows smoking in some public buildings and outdoors. So, this is still a compromise between protecting individual freedoms and the public's health, albeit one that has shifted in favour of the latter (Nuffield Council on Bioethics, 2007, pp 99–117).

Objections

The way of conceiving of public health ethics recommended here is contestable. One objection is that it is overly focused on individuals versus communities, when there are trade-offs between whole communities and sizeable subgroups of people. This kind of problem arises most obviously in multicultural settings. For example, it might be the case that the health of the population can be protected and promoted by requiring a cultural subgroup to desist from a culturally valued practice. But this is not a strong objection to the conception of public health ethics recommended here. In such cases, the cultural subgroup should be thought of as occupying the position of the individual in the problematic triad. Then the same problem arises as before, namely, how the government should adjudicate between the rights and freedoms of a subgroup, on the one hand, and the need to protect and promote the health of the wider population, on the other.

The focus on the role of government as the referee between individuals and communities might be taken to ignore a different kind of public health ethics question, one that begins with individuals and asks after the extent of their obligations and duties to protect and promote population health. How ought an individual to behave when infectious, or a threat to the public's health in some other way? For example, is an individual morally obliged to obtain a vaccination for themself or their child as part of a mass-immunisation programme (Harris and Holm, 1995; Verweij, 2005)?

But again, the conception of public health ethics recommended at the start of this chapter can be defended. In fact, the same problematic triad is encountered here, but described from the perspective of the individual. This is because the questions about the individual's obligations and duties, and whether the government should side with the individual or the community when they clash, are intimately connected. The connection is that the greater the individual's obligations and duties to contribute to the public's health, the greater the justification the government has for siding with communities by protecting and promoting population health at the expense of individual rights and freedoms. And vice versa: the less the individual is obliged, or under a duty, to contribute to the public's health, the less justification the government has for siding with communities by protecting and promoting population health at the expense of individual rights and freedoms.

To illustrate: suppose that an individual is morally obliged to be vaccinated. Then the government is justified in coercing people to get vaccinated by introducing forceful vaccination policies, such as making school enrolment conditional on vaccination status, because in so doing it is simply getting people to fulfil their moral obligations. By contrast, if there is not this moral obligation on individuals to be vaccinated, then the justification for coercive vaccination policies is compromised, because such policies would amount to forcing people to do something they were under no obligation to do.

A more serious rejoinder to the recommended conception of public health ethics is that it is insufficiently radical. There are various versions of this objection, but space here to consider only one in any depth (for a discussion of others, notably that public health ethics should focus on the duties of states to reduce health inequalities within a population, see Holland, 2007, pp x–xii). So far, public health ethics has been conceived in a very ethnocentric way, in that the problematic triad on which it is said to centre arises most obviously in western healthcare contexts such as those of the UK and the US. But the population perspective distinctive of public health should motivate a global health agenda. Otherwise, the "5 and ¾ billion human beings, all of whom we suppose are equal to us [but who are] unaccounted for and indeed unmentioned" (Wikler, 1997, pp 186–7) are being ignored (cf Leon and Walt, 2001; Kass, 2004 pp 237–9). Is the scope of public health ethics as conceived here too parochial and insufficiently global, focusing as it does on a problematic distinctive of western healthcare systems?

There are two points to make in response to this worry. The first is delicate. Because public health invites awareness of the plight of vulnerable people in non-western contexts, it is a way of pursuing an agenda of global health and justice. This is entirely laudable. But public health ethics is a sub-discipline within medical ethics or bioethics and, as such, must centre on and wrestle with ethical problems and dilemmas. Many judgements about global health and justice are ethical, but not ethically problematic, because they are simply correct. For example, consider judgements such as "resources ought to be allocated so as to alleviate public health problems in the developing world" and "it is wrong to increase economic wealth in the north at the expense of the health of people in the south". These are ethical judgements because they contain ethical concepts, but they are not problematic ethical judgements, because no one could present a principled objection to them. This is not to deny that some people in fact do dissent from them; the point is that such dissent is not principled – that is, not the upshot of arguments and considerations that genuinely count against these judgements – but is grounded in apathy or a selfish vested interest in maintaining global inequalities. Since judgements of these kinds are incontestably correct ethical judgements, they cannot be the focus of public health ethics, which should centre on problematic ethical judgements and dilemmas.

Saying that judgements such as "resources ought to be allocated so as to alleviate public health problems in the developing world" are ethically unproblematic could be confused with the claim that such judgements are not problematic at all. Of course, such a judgement is highly problematic, in the sense that actually diverting resources to improve public health in the developing world has proved enormously difficult. But this difficulty is practical; specifically, political, economic and cultural obstacles to meeting an agenda of global health and justice seem difficult to the point of being insurmountable. The point is that the judgement itself is surely ethically non-contentious, even though acting on it is highly problematic. So we can retain public health's role as a focus for a radical agenda of global health and justice without confusing it with public health ethics, conceived as a sub-discipline within medical ethics and bioethics. The two are entirely compatible, the latter in no way inimical to the former.

The second, less contentious, point is that the conception of public health ethics with which this discussion began accommodates much of what has come to be known as developing-world bioethics. To illustrate, in a seminal piece Angell (1997) described clinical trials in third-world contexts that failed to respect the principle of equipoise by denying a proven treatment to placebo control groups. One response is that the trials represent the best way to protect and promote public health, given the specific circumstances of the relevant populations (Resnik, 1998). This is a neat demonstration of the conception of public health ethics set out at the start of this chapter. In this case, the right of individuals to a proven treatment is at odds with the need to protect and promote the health of the population, public health ethics centring on how to adjudicate in such a dispute. In these cases, the recommended conception of public health ethics accommodates the global dimension of public health.

Expansion

Public health ethics as conceived here seems robust. However, there is one strong case for expanding it. The problematic triad described at the outset ignores the fact that each of the main types of public health programme contains distinctive ethical issues. For example, epidemiology is a research programme that presents research ethics issues, some of which are familiar from other research agendas, but others of which – such as appropriate consent to participate, given the longevity and massive data sets typical of epidemiological research projects – are highly distinctive (American College of Epidemiology, 2000). Similarly, screening is an unusual kind of health intervention which, again, introduces distinctive ethical issues, such as the kinds of conditions for which it would be appropriate to screen (National Screening Committee, 1998). The same point applies to mass immunisation and health promotion. For example, a distinctive ethical issue that arises in the former is how to understand and accommodate sincere conscientious objection to vaccines (Hobson-West, 2003); and whether it is morally permissible to employ the techniques of commercial marketing in so-called social marketing is a question raised by health promotion activities aimed at health behaviour changes (Andreasen, 2001).

This suggests a conception of public health ethics somewhat different from that with which this chapter started: not a problematic triad, but a taxonomy of public health interventions and their distinctive ethical components. However, although different, these two ways of conceiving of public health ethics are compatible. So the obvious move is to expand the conception of public health ethics outlined at the start of this chapter – which centres on a problematic triad – with this second way of thinking of public health ethics. And this is what most writers on the subject do, because, typically, the problem of trading off individuals and communities in public health contexts is combined with an ethical evaluation of specific kinds of public health interventions (Holland, 2007). The upshot is that the conception of public health ethics has to be expanded from the problematic triad described at the start of the chapter to include reflection on ethical issues that arise in specific kinds of public health activities.

Summary

The point of this discussion is to recommend a conception of public health ethics. This centres on the problem of how to adjudicate between individual rights and freedoms on the one hand, and protecting and promoting the public's health on the other. Despite various worries about it, this conception has proved robust. However, it needs supplementing, because public health ethics is also about the distinctive ethical issues raised by particular kinds of public health interventions.

How should we do public health ethics?

How should the clash between individual rights and freedoms, on the one hand, and the need to protect and promote the health of the public, on the other, be addressed? What is the best method of analysis for public health ethics?

Rights

One public health ethics methodology employs human rights. The idea is that we can do public health ethics by sorting out the important rights that figure in a public health problem, and then act so as to respect them. There is much to applaud about this. For example, a rights-based approach has the practical intent of protecting and promoting population health, because a way to try to improve public health is by enforcing human (that is, universal) rights in health and healthcare. Addressing public health ethics via human rights sounds promising, and has been advocated by some very influential writers in the field (Mann, 1995; cf Gruskin and Loff, 2002).

But there are serious worries about this rights-based approach. There are notorious conceptual difficulties about rights. "Human rights do not have secure status in contemporary philosophical thinking about social justice" (Wikler, 1997, p 187), and even if they did, rights often conflict with one another in ways that are not at all easily resolved. Advocates of the rights-based approach might retort that this amounts to no more than that more conceptual work on rights is required in order to sort them out and establish their status. But the worry is not just that rights are ambiguous; rather, it seems that the only way to disambiguate rights talk is to determine the obligations enshrined in a right. For example, the only way to interpret 'the right to healthcare' is to determine "*who* has to do *what* for *whom*" (O'Neill, 2002, p 42). This implies that obligations, not rights, are fundamental: "Taking rights as basic to ethics, including health care ethics, does not get close enough to the action" (O'Neill, 2002, p 42), because the action is around ethical obligations, not human rights.

A different conceptual problem with the rights-based approach is that it threatens to merely restate, not resolve, the dilemma at the core of public health ethics, in terms of rights. Suppose the dilemma between individuals and communities is addressed via rights. What kinds of rights might suggest themselves as pertinent? One is the right of communities to be protected from health-threatening behaviours of individuals; another is the right of individuals to, say, privacy. But this is just the original public health ethics problem, expressed in terms of rights. The clash between individuals and communities has been rewritten as the clash between individual rights and communal rights. The terms of the debate have changed, but no progress has been made.

Two lines of thought

If not rights-based, then what kind of methodology is pertinent to public health ethics? Here, two lines of thought will be pursued. They share a structure. Each starts with what seems like a fairly straightforward suggestion as to how to go about public health ethics. In both cases, this straightforward suggestion encounters difficulties. But again in both cases, the original, straightforward suggestion can be adapted and developed into a viable public health methodology. The upshot is two ways of going about public health ethics. The first methodology sketched here is rather general and conceptual, while the second is more focused and practical.

Frameworks

The first line of thought starts with the fairly straightforward suggestion that public health ethics needs a framework (Gostin and Lazzarini, 1997). A number of writers have pursued this. Kass (2001, p 1777) suggests a six-step framework, "an analytic tool, designed to help public health professionals consider the ethics implications of proposed interventions, policy proposals, research initiatives, and programs". Childress et al (2002, p 171) discern "a loose set of general moral considerations – clusters of moral concepts and norms that are variously called values, principles, or rules – that are arguably relevant to public health". They go on to propose five justificatory conditions "to help determine whether promoting public health warrants overriding such values as individual liberty or justice", namely, effectiveness, proportionality, necessity, least infringement, and public justification (p 173).

There is a general problem with this suggestion. Frameworks suggest rigid constructions into which can be shoehorned the discussion of any public health ethics problem. But this is inappropriate, because any framework will carry assumptions about the issues and lines of enquiry important in public health ethics, when public health ethics is a nascent discipline that should be allowed to develop before such assumptions are put in place. Frameworks should emerge out of the practice of public health ethics, not vice versa. Furthermore, public health activities take place in a myriad of contexts that create idiosyncratic ethical challenges. Is it really feasible to think that all these can be fitted into one framework?

To illustrate, Martin (2004) discusses the implications of the severe acute respiratory syndrome (SARS) outbreak for public health policy and practice. She argues that the global nature of such threats necessitates a framework for public heath ethics and goes on to suggest one, based on a focus on what she calls "commonalities":

> For all the differences in economic, historical and cultural development across states, there is significant commonality in their public health systems ... Given such commonality, an agreed global framework is not out of the question. A natural starting point would be for individual states to draft their own public health codes or frameworks, and for these to be drawn together to identify common denominators. (pp 13–14)

The suggested framework is built up around nine claims, each of which describes a commonality, sometimes followed by a caveat acknowledging diversity. The final claim is:

> All public health systems must undertake unpopular tasks which infringe the rights and privacy of individual citizens, such as surveillance, coercion and advocacy, although states may differ in the extent to which they feel justified in these interventions. (p 13)

But this tacitly confirms that frameworks are inappropriate ways of going about public health ethics. Martin is right to say that public health ethics centres on the permissibility of infringements on "the rights and privacy of individual citizens" by the government in order to protect and promote the health of the population. But, given that "states may differ in the extent to which they feel justified in these interventions", there is no commonality here on which to build a shared framework, other than the very problem any suggested framework is constructed to address.

Nonetheless, it would surely be too quick to dismiss altogether the suggestion that frameworks are relevant to public health ethics methodology. A different kind of framework can be envisaged. It should retain the advantages of marshalling public health ethics thinking, but avoid being too rigid for a field as protean as public health. The place to start is by noting that the problematic central to public health ethics – individual versus community – is as old as philosophy itself, albeit that public health is a new context for it. Given this, there must be a wealth of moral and political theory applicable to public health, generated in philosophy by the time-honoured 'individual versus community' problem. How can a philosophically informed framework for reflection on any public health ethics problem be based on these foundations (cf Nijhuis and van der Maesen, 1994)?

Reactions to and reflections on public health interventions are typically based on two major pieces of theory. The first theory is from moral philosophy. Utilitarianism is the moral theory that says that the right action – or, in this case, public health policy intervention – is that which will maximise utility in the form of welfare, well-being or benefit (see Rachels and Rachels, 2007, pp 100–16). Public health is a utilitarian endeavour in that the whole point of public health is to make the world a better place by implementing policies that protect and improve the health of populations. The second theory is from political philosophy. Liberalism (Ryan, 1993) is the political philosophy that provides "a basic moral view on social life; one, moreover, that happens to be dominant in contemporary [western] society" (Zwart, 1999, p 31). As Gostin (2003, p 1141) puts it, it is our *"de facto* political ideology". Although harder to sum up in a slogan, liberalism is distinguished by its emphasis on individual rights and freedoms and, correlatively, its insistence that state interference in the lives of individuals is justified only to avoid harms to third parties.

Utilitarianism and liberalism map neatly onto the central problem in public health ethics. The dilemma between individuals and communities is the clash between the utilitarian public health agenda of maximising population health gain, and the liberal emphasis on individual rights and freedoms. Hence, there is a typical dialectic concerning public health interventions. An intervention is proposed because, from the population perspective, it is expected to maximise utility in the form of public health protection or promotion. But it imposes on individuals by, for example, requiring them to give up some preferred behaviour, forcing them to participate in some risky programme, or invading their privacy.

Individuals respond by invoking the language of liberalism: they resist the intervention because it is an assault on their individual liberties; they have a right to do such-and-such or to decline to do such-and-such, as a matter of personal freedom. Sometimes the liberal objection is so strong that a public health intervention is shelved or withdrawn. Sometimes the utilitarian gains are so promising that individual liberties are sacrificed for them. Whichever way it goes, the debate can be put in the theoretical framework of utilitarianism versus liberalism.

How might this framework be further developed? There is space only to illustrate. Utilitarianism and liberalism, presented here in their most basic forms, have been much discussed and there are far more sophisticated versions of each. So, the framework can be developed by deploying further resources to be found in both theories. For example, so far as public health ethics is concerned, rule-utilitarianism is a more compelling version of utilitarianism than the act-utilitarian view, which considers directly the moral value of public health interventions. For example, the policy of withholding medical treatment from recalcitrant smokers might well maximise utility, so would be justified on direct or act-utilitarian grounds; but not according to rule-utilitarianism, because it is not the case that the rule 'treat according to how patients acquired their condition' would maximise utility (Underwood et al, 1993; Peters and Glanz, 2007).

Likewise, there are resources within liberalism for querying the simple-minded liberal objection that public health interventions are assaults on personal freedoms. Freedom is the concept central to liberalism, but there are different conceptions of freedom. The liberal objection deploys the negative conception of freedom as 'absence of constraint'. But the sophisticated liberal can appeal to positive conceptions of freedom to justify interventions that impinge on freedom negatively construed. For example, coercive public health interventions such as banning smoking in some public places and hard-hitting health communications campaigns are justified as increasing people's effective freedom to live healthily (Swift, 2001, pp 51–68).

Furthermore, moral and political theories that critique utilitarianism and liberalism can be built into the framework. First, there are non-consequentialist moral theories that rival utilitarianism. For example, Kant's deontological, or duty-bound, ethics is based on dictums such as always treat people as ends-in-themselves and never as mere means to ends (Rachels and Rachels, 2007, pp 130–40). This needs building in because of the danger inherent in public health's population perspective of using individuals as means to achieving public health goals. Second, there are anti-liberal political theories that rival liberalism. The best example is communitarianism, a political philosophy based on the forceful criticism that liberalism misconceives people as isolated, atomistic, individual rights bearers when in fact people are essentially communal creatures who are members of valuable communities (Childress and Bernheim, 2003). This needs building into a reflective framework, because it is the political-philosophical corollary to public health's population perspective. (For a more developed construction of a framework along the lines recommended here, see Nuffield Council on Bioethics, 2007).

The construction of this kind of philosophically informed framework for reflection on public health ethics is crucial to the development of the discipline. Without it, public health ethics degenerates into a trade in intuitions about health, freedom, and community. On the other hand, it is an unashamedly academic framework that requires commitment to conceptual work that is usually something of a luxury for public health professionals. Can this framework be combined with another kind of methodology that is less conceptually demanding and more practical?

Public health principlism

Public health ethics is a branch of medical ethics or bioethics. These latter are now well-established disciplines, so a seemingly straightforward suggestion is that the principles and paradigms of medical ethics and bioethics can be borrowed and applied to public health ethics. But there is a subtle difficulty with this. The main achievement of 50 or so years of medical ethics and bioethics is an increased recognition of patients' rights, grounded in greater awareness of their autonomy, which has helped to effect a shift away from medical authoritarianism. For example, the individual's right to consent to medical treatment and participation in medical research – grounded in their ability to decide such matters for themselves – is now well established. But the focus of public health ethics is the dilemma between individual rights and community benefit. So, simply to apply the principles and paradigms of medical ethics and bioethics to public health ethics would be to assume that individual rights have priority over communal benefit, when it is the clash or trade-off between these that is the point of the discussion (Thomas, 2003).

Notwithstanding this difficulty, it is surely extreme to say that disciplines such as medical ethics and bioethics make no methodological contribution to public health ethics. A sensible position is that principles and paradigms of medical ethics and bioethics can be adapted to help resolve public health ethics problems. To illustrate, consider principlism, a familiar and influential methodology well established in medical ethics. Famously, Beauchamp and Childress (2001) defined the four main principles for biomedical ethics as follows:

1. The principle of respect for autonomy: at a minimum, self-rule that is free both from controlling interference by others and from limitations, such as inadequate understanding, that prevent meaningful choice.
2. The principle of beneficence: a moral obligation to act for the benefit of others.
3. The principle of non-maleficence: an obligation not to inflict harm on others.
4. The principle of justice: fair, equitable, and appropriate treatment in light of what is due or owed to persons.

Arguably, none of these principles is applicable to public health ethics, for reasons already encountered. Invoking the principle of autonomy amounts to simply opting for the individual against the community, which is clearly no way to resolve the dilemma between individuals and communities (Horner, 2000, p 50). The problem with applying the other three principles arose in the previous discussion of rights. It threatens to merely restate, not resolve, the dilemma between individuals and communities. In other words, this dilemma can be restated in terms of Beauchamp and Childress's principles of beneficence, non-maleficence and justice, respectively, as follows. Whose *benefit* should be prioritised: that of the individual or their community? Which *evil* or *harm* should be attended to: the harm of transgressing individual rights, or the harm done to communities when individuals act self-interestedly? Is *justice* best served by allowing individuals their freedoms, or by imposing on individuals for the sake of the population as a whole?

It turns out that "the straightforward application of the principles of autonomy, beneficence, non-maleficence and justice in public health practice is problematic" (Upshur, 2002, p 101). But simply to abandon principlism would be a shame, because it is well suited to alerting non-philosophical professionals to the ethical dimension of their speciality, and it is practical and flexible. Better, then, to adapt principlism by developing principles better suited to public health. Upshur (2002) does this, suggesting the following public health ethics principles. John Stuart Mill's *harm principle* presents a general condition on restrictions by government on the liberty of an individual or group:

the only purpose for which power can be rightfully exercised over any member of a civilised community, against his will, is to prevent harm to others. His own good, either physical or moral, is not a sufficient warrant. (Mill, 1975, pp 14–15)

The principle of *least restrictive or coercive means* ushers in a list of ways of intervening to achieve public health goals, in order of ethical preference from less to more coercive. Upshur (2002, p 102) suggests the following list: "Education, facilitation, and discussion should precede interdiction, regulation or incarceration."

The *reciprocity principle* is based on the fact that compliance with public health requirements can be burdensome for individuals. Where so, there are obligations on public health bodies to provide the means to enable individuals to comply – such as relevant information – and to compensate individuals for the cost of their compliance with public health measures: "Society must be prepared to facilitate individuals and communities in their efforts to discharge their duties" (Upshur, 2002, p 173).

The *transparency* principle puts various conditions on the process by which public health decisions are made. All stakeholders should be involved, all should have equal input into deliberations, decision making should be clear and transparent, and it should be as free as possible from political and non-political vested interest.

Following Upshur's lead, other principles could serve to help address public health ethics problems. One is the precautionary principle, a statement of which is:

Where there are threats of serious or irreversible damage, lack of full scientific certainty shall not be used as a reason for postponing cost-effective measures to prevent environmental degradation. (United Nations, 1992)

The role of the precautionary principle in public health is under discussion (Wynia, 2005). As Bayer and Fairchild (2004, p 490) comment, "the precautionary principle has implicitly guided public health interventions designed to limit or forestall epidemic outbreak".

Of course, there is much more work to be done in clarifying and refining the principles relevant to public health, but public health principlism is very promising because it is a relatively accessible and practical way of doing public health ethics. The principles play two roles in the analysis of a public health dilemma. First, adverting to the principles can elucidate a dilemma. In other words, applying the principles such as transparency and reciprocity will help to clarify the nature of the dilemma in question. For example, the problem might be that a proposed intervention is more coercive than necessary or would incur costs to individuals that are uncompensated. Second, the principles will help to resolve the dilemma. In any particular case, one or more of the principles will be the most pertinent, so it will be reasonable to resolve the problem by abiding by them. For example, it might be the case that a public health initiative is dubious because its epidemiological basis is questionable, in which case the precautionary principle can be invoked.

Concluding remarks

The first part of this chapter presented a conception of public health ethics as centring on trade-offs between individual rights and population health benefits. This was defended and augmented. The second part of the chapter suggested two ways of going about public health ethics. The first is to construct a philosophically informed reflective framework, the second is public health principlism. These methodologies are compatible with one another, so they can be pursued in tandem, without needing to choose one at the expense of the other, and they are not exhaustive, so others can be employed alongside them. Crucially, neither these nor any other methodology provide neat answers to public health dilemmas. Rather, they are ways of presenting and refining the kind of ongoing rigorous arguments that ought to comprise public health ethics.

References

American College of Epidemiology (2000) 'Ethics guidelines', *Annals of Epidemiology*, vol 10, no 8, pp 487–97.

Andreasen, A. (ed) (2001) *Ethics in social marketing*, Washington, DC: Georgetown University Press.

Angell, M. (1997) 'The ethics of clinical research in the third world', *The New England Journal of Medicine*, vol 337, no 12, pp 847–9.

Bayer, R. and Fairchild, A. (2004) 'The genesis of public health ethics', *Bioethics*, vol 18, no 6, pp 473–92.

Beauchamp, T. and Childress, J. (2001) *Principles of biomedical ethics* (5th edn), Oxford: Oxford University Press.

Childress, J. and Bernheim, R. (2003) 'Beyond the liberal and communitarian impasse: a framework and vision for public health', *Florida Law Review*, vol 55, no 5, pp 1191–219.

Childress, J., Faden, R., Gaare, R., Gostin, L., Kahn, J., Bonnie, R., Kass, N., Mastroianni, A., Moreno, J. and Nieburg, P. (2002) 'Public health ethics: mapping the terrain', *Journal of Law, Medicine and Ethics*, vol 30, no 2, pp 170–8.

Gostin, L. (2003) 'When terrorism threatens health: how far are limitations on personal and economic liberties justified?', *Florida Law Review*, vol 55, no 5, pp 1105–69.

Gostin, L. and Lazzarini, Z. (1997) *Human rights and public health in the AIDS pandemic*, Oxford: Oxford University Press.

Gruskin, S. and Loff, B. (2002) 'Do human rights have a role in public health work?', *The Lancet*, vol 360, no 9348, p 1880.

Harris, J. and Holm, S. (1995) 'Is there a moral obligation not to infect others?', *British Medical Journal*, vol 311, no 7014, pp 1215–17.

Hobson-West, P. (2003) 'Understanding vaccination resistance: moving beyond risk', *Health, Risk and Society*, vol 5, no 3, pp 273–83.

Holland, S. (2007) *Public health ethics*, Cambridge: Polity Press.

Horner, J. (2000) 'For debate. The virtuous public health physician', *Journal of Public Health Medicine*, vol 22, no 1, pp 48–53.

Kass, N. (2001) 'An ethics framework for public health', *American Journal of Public Health*, vol 91, no 11, pp 1776–82.

Kass, N. (2004) 'Public health ethics: from foundations and frameworks to justice and global public health', *Journal of Law, Medicine and Ethics*, vol 32, no 2, pp 232–42.

Leon, D. and Walt, G. (eds) (2001) *Poverty, inequality and health: An international perspective*, Oxford: Oxford University Press.

Mann, J. (1995) 'Human rights and the new public health', *Health and Human Rights*, vol 1, no 3, pp 229–33.

Martin, R. (2004) 'Public health ethics and SARS: seeking an ethical framework to global public health governance', *Law, Social Justice and Global Development*, vol 1 (e-journal, www2.warwick.ac.uk/fac/soc/law/elj/lgd/2004_1/martin/).

Mill, J.S. (1975) 'On liberty', in J.S. Mill, *Three essays: On liberty, representative government, the subjection of women*, Oxford: Oxford University Press, pp 5–141.

National Screening Committee (1998) *First report of the National Screening Committee*, London: Health Departments of the United Kingdom. Available at: www.dh.gov.uk/en/Publicationsandstatistics/Publications/PublicationsPolicyAndGuidance/DH_4006774 (accessed 25 August 2008).

Nijhuis, H. and van der Maesen, L. (1994) 'The philosophical foundations of public health: an invitation to debate', *Journal of Epidemiology and Community Health*, vol 48, no 1, pp 1–3.

Nuffield Council on Bioethics (2007) *Public health: Ethical issues*, London: Nuffield Council on Bioethics.

O'Neill, O. (2002) 'Public health or clinical ethics: thinking beyond borders', *Ethics and International Affairs*, vol 16, no 2, pp 35–45.

Peters, M.J. and Glantz, L. (2007) 'Should smokers be refused surgery?', *British Medical Journal*, no 33406 (7583), pp 20–1.

Rachels, J. and Rachels, S. (2007) *The elements of moral philosophy* (5th edn), Boston, MA: McGraw-Hill, ch 8.

Resnik, D. (1998) 'The ethics of HIV research in developing nations', *Bioethics*, vol 12, no 4, pp 286–306.

Ryan, A. (1993) 'Liberalism', in R. Goodin and P. Pettit (eds) *A companion to contemporary political philosophy*, Oxford: Blackwell Publishers, pp 291–311.

Swift, A. (2001) *Political philosophy: A beginners' guide for students and politicians*, Cambridge: Polity Press.

Thomas, J.C. (2003) 'Teaching ethics in schools of public health', *Public Health Reports*, vol 118, pp 279–86.

Underwood, M.J., Bailey, J.S., Shiu, M., Higgs, R. and Garfield, J. (1993) 'Should smokers be offered coronary bypass surgery?', *British Medical Journal*, vol 306 (6884), pp 1047–50.

United Nations (1992) *Report of the United Nations Conference on the Environment and Development (Rio de Janeiro June 3–14) Annex I: Rio Declaration on Environment and Development*, New York: United Nations General Assembly, A/CONF.151/26 (Vol I), Principle 15.

Upshur, R. (2002) 'Principles for the justification of public health intervention', *Canadian Journal of Public Health*, vol 93, no 2, pp 101–3.

Verweij, M. (2005) 'Obligatory precautions against infection', *Bioethics*, vol 19, no 4, pp 323–35.

Wikler, D. (1997) 'Presidential address: bioethics and social responsibility', *Bioethics*, vol 11, no 3–4, pp 185–92.

Wynia, M. (2005) 'Public health principlism: the precautionary principle and beyond', *The American Journal of Bioethics*, vol 5, no 3, pp 3–4.

Zwart, H. (1999) 'All you need is health. Liberal and communitarian views on the allocation of health care resources', in M. Parker (ed) *Ethics and community in the health care professions*, London: Routledge, pp 30–46.

Part Two
Ethics and public health practice

FOUR

What does it mean to 'know' a disease? The tragedy of XDR-TB

Ross Upshur

This chapter explores the classic dilemma faced by public health policy in the face of attempting to control an outbreak of an infectious disease, and how to 'manage' individuals who are infected with the disease – in this case, XDR-TB – in order to protect the population. In other words, the debate focuses on the autonomy of the individual and the legitimate powers of the state to quarantine individuals against their will.

Introduction

Although unpalatable to consider, we are at a watershed in the history of the control of tuberculosis (Fauci, 2007). The progressive increase of resistance of tuberculosis (TB) to pharmacotherapy has raised the possibility of a response to tuberculosis without medications, in essence returning us to the situation as it was in the 19th century or, as some have posited, the dawn of the post-antibiotic age (Raviglione, 2006). The combination of high rates of TB infection with high seropositivity rates for HIV in sub-Saharan Africa has raised the ante of global tuberculosis control.

It is instructive to note that from almost any perspective, tuberculosis is one of the most well-understood diseases in all of medicine. Understanding tuberculosis has been important historically, in constituting the very notion of causality in biology and medicine. Robert Koch explained the concept of infectious diseases and stated his famous postulates largely on the basis of the study of tuberculosis. Our concept of clinical causality is rooted in randomised clinical trials, of which one of the first and most influential was the UK Medical Research Council's streptomycin trial for the treatment of tuberculosis (MRC, 1948). From Hippocrates to the present day, much of our understanding of clinical medicine, bedside lore, and the signs, symptoms and phenomenology of disease arise from our collective experience of tuberculosis.

Knowledge of the disease is extensive in a multitude of dimensions (Verma et al, 2004). We know its genetic fingerprints and its mechanism of resistance at the molecular level. The social determinants of the disease, rooted in poverty, adverse living conditions, and social disadvantage, are not contested (Benatar, 2001). The social consequences of stigma and how these vary from culture to culture are also well characterised (Croft and Croft, 1998; Rajeswari et al, 1999; Khan et al, 2000). There are ample literary allusions to the impact of tuberculosis on human life in the writings of Mann, Dickens, and Dostoyevsky. The opera *La Bohème* and Susan Sontag's *Illness as metaphor* (a significant work of literary criticism) feature tuberculosis prominently (Sontag, 2001). Paleoarcheology has shown that tuberculosis has long been part of the human condition, as witnessed in the bones of mummies. Thus, human interaction with the tuberculosis bacillus is long and devoid of mystery. Few other diseases can claim such abundance of human expression and understanding. Ubiquitous diseases of modernity such as obesity, hypertension or cardiovascular disease can lay no such claim to accumulated science and art.

We know tuberculosis well indeed, yet knowing seems not to matter in terms of increased control. Tuberculosis has transformed from a curable illness in the 1970s and 1980s to a difficult-to-treat-but-still-manageable condition with the emergence of multiple drug-resistant tuberculosis (MDR-TB), followed by the World Health Organization's (WHO) declaration of a global emergency in tuberculosis control in the early 1990s (WHO, 2007). Now, the new millennium witnesses the emergence of extensively drug-resistant tuberculosis (XDR-TB), which may prove to be untreatable (Iseman, 2007a).

The situation is, of course, considerably worse in situations of high TB and HIV burdens. An outbreak in Kwa Zulu-Natal reported in 2006 demonstrated that the synergy between resistant TB and HIV is particularly deadly. The initial report granted XDR-TB membership in an exclusive club of particularly deadly pathogens alongside rabies and Ebola virus (Gandhi et al, 2006).

These trends are bitter news for those wedded to notions of medical progress and the efficacy of knowledge to control disease. Worse still is the recognition that XDR-TB is largely a human creation, and partly the result of the treatment itself. Pillay and Sturm (2007) demonstrated what many thought to be the case all along, that directly observed therapy for tuberculosis (DOTS) contributes to the development of drug resistance. As Iseman argues in the accompanying editorial, the development of XDR-TB is the predictable and logical consequence of treating TB in the first place (Iseman, 2007b). This merely underscores the existential tragedy that is unfolding. Many lament the squandering of useful antibiotics, yet a peculiar silence reigns over the fate of those no longer treatable.

Responding to drug-resistant tuberculosis is perhaps one of the most profound ethical challenges facing global health. One reason for the overarching importance of tuberculosis is that the creation of drug resistance is one of human agency and human failure. Drug-resistant tuberculosis is not the result of catastrophic natural forces such as earthquakes, tsunamis and hurricanes. It is not caused by malign human intent, as are terrorism and war; nor is it fostered by our dysfunctional relationship with the animal kingdom, as are SARS and avian influenza. The locus of risk and control is entirely within the human domain. Our reaction to the emergence of drug-resistant tuberculosis is profoundly ethical, as it raises issues of how justice and human rights are realised in our collective response to a disease.

If we are without effective vaccines or medications to respond to tuberculosis, how should public health systems respond? What is the role of the use of non-therapeutic measures, such as restriction and detention? What are the ethical issues raised by these measures for public health? In what follows, a set of critical questions to the current tuberculosis problematic will be posed by considering three cases of the public health management of drug-resistant tuberculosis. Then an analytic framework evolved with a specific focus on analysing the legitimate use of restrictive measures for the control of tuberculosis will be described.

Case 1 – Andrew Speaker[1]

In May 2007, Andrew Speaker, a personal injury lawyer from Atlanta, Georgia in the US, deliberately plotted a course of travel to avoid reporting to public health authorities. Although this case received extensive publicity, the salient features are important. This gentleman, with documented diagnosed drug-resistant tuberculosis and posing a potential threat of transmission to others, acted in such a way as to avoid detention from duly constituted public health authorities. He left the US, travelled extensively by plane through Europe and, when asked to report to public health authorities in Italy, arranged his flights home to avoid detection by US Immigration Services. However, when he subsequently returned to the US, he was detained under the federal quarantine statutes.

Speaker himself is precisely the sort of individual not associated with tuberculosis. Well educated and resourced, of a high socio-economic status and knowledgeable about legal issues, it still remains unclear as to how he contracted tuberculosis. He found it easy to avoid detection and relatively easy to resist or ignore orders from public health authorities. The ease with which he crossed borders to return to the US posed significant concerns and exposed vulnerabilities regarding how diseases can cross borders without detection.

In this case, fortune was on Speaker's side. When taken to the National Jewish Medical and Research Center in Denver, Colorado, subsequent cultures indicated that he did not in fact have XDR-TB. The general zeitgeist response that it was 'only' MDR-TB should be resisted, as MDR-TB is still a disease associated with high morbidity and mortality. Speaker was fortunate not simply because he had MDR-TB, not XDR-TB, but because his condition was amenable to surgical cure, which is what occurred in his case. He had a lobectomy, which removed all elements of his tuberculosis infection, and he was able to return to his normal life. That he inconvenienced many people and became a highly criticised individual should not detract from the fact that his case raises salient issues about the use of public health measures to control communicable diseases.

Case 2 – Robert Daniels[2]

Daniels is a Russian-American citizen who contracted tuberculosis while living in Russia. He returned to Arizona in the US to seek better healthcare. The details of his case were less publicised than were those of Speaker's. However, what is important in his case is that he refused to comply with public health authorities' orders to act in such a way as not to transmit infections while in public. Specifically, he refused to wear a mask to prevent the spread of respiratory secretions in public. When public health authorities were made aware of this, he was subsequently detained under a court order and placed in a prison cell where he was denied access to communication technologies and kept under video surveillance and bright lights for 24 hours a day. His case drew the attention of civil liberties activists, who regarded his detention as a violation of basic civil rights.

Case 3 – South Africa

In South Africa, high rates of HIV/AIDS are creating a deadly synergy in combination with drug-resistant tuberculosis. The initial report of drug-resistant tuberculosis from Tugula Ferry in Kwa Zulu-Natal indicated 52 of 53 HIV-positive patients and healthcare workers dying within weeks of diagnosis (Gandhi et al, 2006). There was evidence of extensive person-to-person spread and very quickly it has become clear that drug-resistant tuberculosis, particularly MDR and XDR, is extensively endemic in sub-Saharan Africa, particularly in South Africa, with cases reported in most jurisdictions of the country (Ford, 2007). In order to contain the epidemic, South African health authorities have used hospital-based treatment, including mandatory detention. Resistance to the use of hospital treatment has occurred, including well-documented cases of patients absconding from hospital treatment and taking refuge in the community while still infectious. South African police have been used to search for absconders and return them to hospital.

Critical questions

Certainly, individual liberty and human rights must be weighed against risk of harm to communities. However, from the perspective of the mandate and mission of public health, the protection of the public from harm, particularly preventable harm from known infectious diseases, is an overarching moral and legal imperative. The spectre of XDR-TB raises several critical questions that require urgent attention. The questions can be set as follows:

- What is the appropriate level of respect for autonomy and choice when persons harbour untreatable or potentially untreatable communicable diseases?
- Should voluntary measures be the default, and only countermanded with evidence of failure?
- What is the legitimate scope for the use of restrictive measures for communicable disease control?
- What parameters should be placed around the use of restrictive measures? How should these restrictive measures be monitored and evaluated?

One issue is how to manage individuals who are infected and pose a risk to others and are either unable or unwilling to act in such ways as to mitigate exposure. There is clearly a role for the use of involuntary measures in such circumstances. In most constitutional democracies, there are public health laws that provide public health authorities with the ability to detain individuals deemed at risk of spreading disease in the community. As the case examples show, these powers are variably employed and their general effectiveness is unclear. More important for this analysis is that legal and ethical legitimacy are distinct, and the latter does not necessarily follow from the former.

In what follows, a framework for assessing the ethical legitimacy concerning the use of restrictive measures is outlined (Upshur, 2002). In general, it is argued that there are four ethical conditions that need to be considered in the use of restrictive measures for communicable disease control. For reasons of philosophical purity, these principles are not supposed to be analogous to the principlist framework of Beauchamp and Childress (2001). Rather, they serve as heuristics to critically examine the justification for restriction and to evaluate the impact of restriction. The four considerations are: the harm principle, proportionality or use of least restrictive means, reciprocity, and transparency.

Harm principle

This principle derives from J.S. Mill, who writes:

> that the only purpose for which power can be rightfully exercised over any member of the civilised community against his will is to prevent harm to others. His own good, either physical or moral, is not sufficient warrant. He cannot rightfully be compelled to do or forebear because it will be better for him to do so, because it will make him happier, because in the opinion of others, to do so would be wise or even right. The only part of the conduct of anyone for which he is amenable to society is that which concerns others. In the part which merely concerns himself, his independence is of right, absolute. (Mill, 1959)

The harm principle is applicable in the case of XDR or MDR tuberculosis because predictable harm is likely to occur for individuals who are untreated, non-adherent or who are acting in a way such as to not prevent the spread of the disease to others. There is considerable variability in the extent of spread to others from an individual with active tuberculosis. Environmental factors and living conditions play a crucial role in the extent of spread associated with a tuberculosis infection (Reichler et al, 2002). Drug-sensitive tuberculosis disease is amenable to treatment and cure, and exposure to drug-sensitive tuberculosis is amenable to prophylactic treatment. However, no such prophylaxis is available for drug-resistant strains, because they are by definition resistant to those drugs that one would use for prophylaxis of disease.

Some subtleties of tuberculosis are relevant to the discussion of the harm principle. The vast majority of tuberculosis infections are latent infections. This means that individuals harbour tuberculosis bacteria in their bodies, but their immune systems keep the infection in check. They are not capable of spreading the disease to others and therefore pose no harm to others. Tuberculosis causes a wide range of manifestations of disease, including pulmonary (in the respiratory system) and extra-pulmonary (in the bones, or other systems such as the kidneys). Individuals with extra-pulmonary tuberculosis, like those with latent infections, cannot spread the disease to others, no matter how severe their illness. Only pulmonary tuberculosis can be spread from person to person, via coughing or sneezing the tubercle bacillus into the ambient atmosphere, and there must be sufficient bacteria in the sputum (smear positivity) to pose a hazard to others.

Hence, only smear-positive individuals with tuberculosis in communities are a risk to others, with the predictable consequence of increased infection and disease and, in those vulnerable populations, death. In the case of tuberculosis, there are increased risks of transmission and illness to healthcare providers themselves, adding a further dimension of complexity to the problem (Joshi et al, 2006). Therefore, on any grounds considered, individuals with smear-positive XDR or MDR tuberculosis may pose harm to communities, and thus the harm principle would be satisfied, indicating the possible need for restrictive measures.

Least restrictive means

Proportionality is an important value in the response to tuberculosis. In constitutional democracies, individuals are protected from needless coercion from powerful bodies such as state-empowered public health authorities. Any restrictions on fundamental liberties or protected human rights (particularly mobility rights) need to be legal, legitimate and necessary, and applied only by those with legitimate authority.

This reasoning supports use of the least restrictive measures necessary for achieving public health ends. This means that education and facilitation are preferred to interdiction and incarceration. However, it is not necessary that failure of lesser means must be demonstrated before the use of more restrictive measures in all cases. If one can persuade an individual with drug-resistant tuberculosis to voluntarily curtail their activities in the community and reduce the risk of exposure to others, and this can be monitored and adjudicated in a sufficiently sophisticated way, this may suffice. However, if there is evidence of failure of voluntary means, more restrictive measures are clearly justified, up to and including involuntary hospitalisation or detention orders.

Worsening drug resistance could potentially render consideration of less restrictive means moot, because if there is no effective treatment, there is not a set of graduated lesser restrictive means to be considered by public health authorities. The acceptability of the means of addressing drug-resistant tuberculosis, however, is an important consideration for community dialogue. Freedom of movement may be an acceptable sacrifice to both individuals and communities. Consideration of enforced therapy would be more problematic, as it has little ethical support.

Reciprocity

In terms of the reciprocity principle it is important to recognise that individuals with diseases such as tuberculosis are not criminals. They are suffering from a serious illness and require care and support in order to return to health, if achievable, and palliation of symptoms if no return to good health is possible. If the incentives of the social service sector and healthcare system militate against individuals acting in such a way as not to infect others there is no clear incentive to act in such a way as not to endanger others (Singh et al, 2007). For example, in the South African situation, cutting off social benefits to individuals who are hospitalised puts family members who are dependent on those benefits at risk. This is particularly so in cases where the individual tuberculosis patient requiring in-hospital treatment is the chief breadwinner of the family or the one whose social benefits provide the means of income and survival for the family.

Quite clearly, there is a requirement on behalf of society to provide incentives and a sufficiently humane and dignified context of care for individuals to discharge their duties to society. In essence, by invoking restrictive measures we are asking individuals to curtail their movements largely for the public good. The individual benefit of giving up such rights is minimal.

Harris and Holm (1995) outline the idea that there is a duty not to harm others by virtue of communicating diseases. They argue that the moral duty to behave responsibly and not knowingly put other people at risk is not a duty confined simply to infections that have life-threatening implications. They state:

> It is a duty which all people with communicable diseases
> have. It is, however, also a duty which we can expect [them]
> to discharge only if they live in a community that does not
> leave them with all the burdens involved in discharging
> that duty. (p 1217)

This is referred to here as the infectious disease reciprocity condition. That is, if public health authorities wish to invoke restrictive measures, they must, in a reciprocal manner, provide assistance and enable individuals to discharge those duties. Part of this obligation is providing appropriate protections for them while they are hospitalised. Part of the obligation is also working with communities in order that they understand that individuals must sacrifice constitutionally guaranteed liberties in order to reduce the risk of infection.

Reciprocity is one of the key issues in infectious disease and public health ethics. The question becomes one of establishing and specifying exactly who has the responsibility for providing for those whose liberties are restricted. This cannot be resolved in this present discussion, but is an important question for future research in public health ethics.

Discourse ethics

Finally, all the conditions previously discussed indicate the need for concern with the fairness of discourse, and here discourse ethics is used as a means to move forward. When contemplating the use of restrictive measures, it is important that individuals whose rights are going to be abrogated have representation or voice. It is also important that there be a forum (not necessarily a court of law) wherein all participants have equal say and fair representation, that all power differentials are negated, and that all who participate in discourse have equal chances to present interpretations, make assertions, recommendations, explanations and corrections. Finally, there must be some mechanism by which these decisions are appealed.

Part of the concern for including discourse ethics in outlining the ethical legitimacy of restrictive measures relates to what has been called judicial deference in public health decision making (Reis, 2007). In Canada, the legal tradition finds resoundingly in favour of public health authorities when it comes to adjudicating and deciding upon orders for detention of individuals who pose risk to communities. Judicial deference gives public health authorities considerable latitude in terms of scope and application of detention orders. Thus, necessary checks and balances need to be in place, and given that historically courts have been found to be overly deferential to public health authorities, it might be of value to create an independent tribunal to adjudicate these discussions. Models of such independent tribunals exist, particularly in the field of psychiatric care. Those individuals who have been found guilty by virtue of diminished capacity are reviewed on a periodic basis by an independent tribunal, which includes medical experts, lawyers and community members. A well-constituted tribunal would be an ideal forum to hear discussions about the duration and conditions of detention.

Application of framework

The framework previously outlined serves as a point of departure for addressing the questions posed. The framework addresses the question of whether, in fact, a justification exists for the use of restrictive measures for the control of diseases such as tuberculosis. Individuals with smear-positive drug-resistant pulmonary tuberculosis who fail to comply with therapy do pose a threat to communities. If they fail voluntary measures, there is a strong prima facie argument for the use of restrictive measures. However, the framework does not give unfettered power to the state to detain individuals in any way in which it sees fit, for whatever purpose.

Observing the concepts of reciprocity and discourse ethics places an obligation on those arguing for restrictive measures to outline the acceptability of the conditions under which the individuals will be kept. The fora or tribunals are discourse spaces where the adequacy of these arrangements can be adjudicated and contested. In this way, one can argue for the legitimacy of restrictive measures separate from the acceptability and legitimacy of the conditions of restriction.

Therefore, looking back at the cases identified, it was both legally and ethically justified to detain both Speaker and Daniels. However, the manner in which Mr Daniels was detained failed to meet minimal standards and should be criticised, and the individuals who kept him under such circumstances should be held accountable and appropriate consequences determined to redress the wrongs done. Mr Speaker, on the other hand, was treated appropriately and detained in a humane, dignified way, despite the amount of adverse publicity he suffered.

More troubling however, is the situation evolving in South Africa. There are already more cases of MDR- and XDR-TB than there are beds to provide care. Individuals have waited for treatment in the community while still symptomatic, and spread the disease while waiting for hospital treatment. In this context, restrictive measures may have little effect, and detaining individuals by law once they have been hospitalised, after they have been in the community for extensive periods of time, seems somewhat wrongheaded. There was one report in 2007 of an individual with tuberculosis being shot in a demonstration outside a healthcare facility in Johannesburg.

In South Africa, the conditions of reciprocity have not been met, and the social incentives have not been realigned to make the pursuit of treatment for drug-resistant tuberculosis a dominant strategy. In fact, a very difficult stage is being reached where the disincentives for treatment may far outweigh any incentives, particularly when it seems that treatment for XDR-TB may be futile. In that case, disease will be driven back into communities, and the issue there is how to make communities safe from, but also willing to accept, individuals with drug-resistant tuberculosis in their midst. There is always the residual fear of vigilantism, which was a prominent feature of responses of some communities to other communities with smallpox (Barbera et al, 2001). There is a fine line to be trodden in promoting communities' acceptance of individuals with diseases that pose harm. While it may be within the realm of acceptable practice for family members willingly to accept exposure, there is a strong likelihood that many other individuals may have an aversion to this possibility, an aversion which may have unfortunate consequences for individuals with tuberculosis. Tuberculosis is and has been a highly stigmatised illness (Battin et al, 2006) that still generates fear in communities.

One of the most important horizons in public health ethics is trying to envision how to build communities that are regarded as tuberculosis friendly. This will not occur overnight. However, while the world is adjusting to the new realities of drug-resistant tuberculosis and contemplating the possibility of a future with completely drug-resistant tuberculosis, it is imperative that the manner in which the illness is conceptualised and managed in the first place be rethought. It is particularly important that responses to tuberculosis do not worsen already existing disadvantage (Gostin and Powers, 2006). It is important that the public health dimensions of tuberculosis illness be incorporated into the tuberculosis patient's bill of rights. As it stands right now, it is very unclear in stating what, if any, obligations individuals with tuberculosis have, specifically with regard to acting responsibly and not knowingly transmitting illness to others. It is important to communicate to individuals with tuberculosis that failure to adhere to therapy may result in the generation of drug-resistant strains, with the attendant concerns of untreatability. How many courses of therapy are possible, particularly for any given individual, may need to be articulated, especially in light of the development of worsening resistance (Macklin, 2006). In this case, it may be necessary to indicate to individuals at the outset that failure to adhere or the development of resistance may result in active therapy with curative intent being stopped, and that palliation may be the only option for them.

In conclusion, the emergence of XDR-TB is a dystopian moment in history. What is an extremely well-known disease is now on the verge of becoming a rare event – a truly curable illness becoming incurable, with the incalculable impact this would have on communities, health services, systems and individuals globally. It is time for sober reflection on the limits of positivistic scientific approaches to the solution to this problem, and perhaps it is time to embrace an agency that more holistically and emphatically embraces interventions based on the broader determinants of health.

Until that time, there is no doubt a role for the use of restrictive measures to prevent the spread of such diseases in communities. Although not palatable in the eyes of many, especially those with high regard for civil liberties, the good of the community likely outweighs any concern for individual liberties in these extreme cases.

Notes
[1] For more details see 'TB patient asked to testify before Senate'. Available at: http://abcnews.go.com/GMA/story?id=3249254&page=1 (accessed 27 August 2008).

[2] For more details see 'Drug-resistant TB strain raises ethical dilemma. Man locked up indefinitely, sparking civil liberties debate'. Available at: www.msnbc.msn.com/id/17915965/wid/11915773/-44k (accessed 27 August 2008).

References
Barbera, S., MacIntyre, A., Gostin, L., Inglesby, T., O'Toole, T., DeAtley, C., Tonat, K. and Layton, M. (2001) 'Large-scale quarantine following biological terrorism in the United States scientific examination, logistic and legal limits, and possible consequences', *Journal of the American Medical Association*, vol 286, no 21, pp 2711–17.

Battin, M., Francis, L., Smith, C. and Jacobson, J. (2006) 'The patient as victim and vector: challenge of infectious disease', in R. Rhodes, L. Francis and A. Silvers (eds) *The Blackwell guide to medical ethics*, Oxford and New York: Blackwell, ch 15.

Beauchamp, T. and Childress, J. (2001) *Principles of biomedical ethics* (5th edn), Oxford: Oxford University Press.

Benatar, S. (2001) 'Respiratory health in a globalizing world', *American Journal of Respiratory Critical Care Medicine*, vol 163, no 5, pp 1064–7.

Croft, R. and Croft, R. (1998) 'Expenditure and loss of income incurred by tuberculosis patients before reaching effective treatment in Bangladesh', *International Journal Tuberculosis and Lung Disease*, vol 2, no 3, pp 252–4.

Fauci, A. (2007) *Action now can halt new TB strains*, TB Alliance – Global alliance for TB drug development. Available at: http://new.tballiance.org/newscenter/view-innews.php?id=655 (accessed 27 August 2008).

Ford, N. (2007) 'Highlights from the 38th Union Conference on Lung Health', *Lancet Infectious Diseases*, vol 7, no 12, p 767.

Gandhi, N., Moll, A., Sturm, A., Pawinski, R., Govender, T., Lalloo, U., Zeller, K., Andrews, J. and Friedland, G. (2006) 'Extensively drug-resistant tuberculosis as a cause of death in patients co-infected with tuberculosis and HIV in a rural area of South Africa', *Lancet*, vol 368, no 9547, pp 1575–80.

Gostin, L. and Powers, M. (2006) 'What does social justice require for the public's health? Public health ethics and policy imperatives', *Health Affairs*, vol 25, no 4, pp 1053–60.

Harris, J. and Holm, S. (1995) 'Is there a moral obligation not to infect others?' *BMJ*, vol 311, no 7014, pp 1215–7.

Iseman, M. (2007a) 'Extensively drug-resistant Mycobacterium tuberculosis: Charles Darwin would understand', *Clinical Infectious Diseases*, vol 45, no 11, pp 1415–6.

Iseman, M. (2007b) *XDR-TB, AIDS, and the future of TB control – An apocalyptic tale*. Available at: www.uchsc.edu/ccfar/docs/MichaelIsemanKeynoteSpeakerPresentation.pdf (accessed 27 August 2008).

Joshi, R., Reingold, A., Menzies, D. and Pai, M. (2006) 'Tuberculosis among health-care workers in low- and middle-income countries: a systematic review', *PLoS Medicine*, vol 3, no 12, e494.

Khan, A., Walley, J., Newell, J. and Imdad, N. (2000) 'Tuberculosis in Pakistan: socio-cultural constraints and opportunities in treatment', *Social Science and Medicine*, vol 50, no 2, pp 247–54.

Macklin, R. (2006) 'No shortage of dilemmas: comment on "They call it 'patient selection' in Khayelitsha"', *Cambridge Quarterly of Healthcare Ethics*, vol 15, no 3, pp 313–21.

Mill, J.S. (1959) 'On liberty', in B. Wishy (ed) *Prefaces to liberty: Selected writings*, Lanham, MD: University Press.

MRC (Medical Research Council) (1948) 'Streptomycin treatment of pulmonary tuberculosis', *British Medical Journal*, vol 2, pp 769–82.

Pillay, M. and Sturm, A. (2007) 'Evolution of the extensively drug-resistant F15/LAM4/KZN strain of Mycobacterium tuberculosis in KwaZulu-Natal, South Africa', *Clinical Infectious Diseases*, vol 45, no 11, pp 1409–14.

Rajeswari, R., Balasubramanian, R., Muniyandi, M., Geetharamani, S., Thresa, X. and Venkatesan, P. (1999) 'Socio-economic impact of tuberculosis on patients and family in India', *International Journal of Tuberculosis and Lung Disease*, vol 3, no 10, pp 869–77.

Raviglione, M. (2006) 'XDR-TB: entering the post-antibiotic era?', *International Journal of Tuberculosis and Lung Disease*, vol 10, no 11, pp 1185–7.

Reichler, M., Reves, R., Bur, S., Thompson, V., Mangura, B., Ford, J., Valway, S. and Onorato, I. (2002) 'Evaluation of investigations conducted to detect and prevent transmission of tuberculosis', *Journal of the American Medical Association*, vol 287, no 8, pp 991–5.

Reis, N. (2007) 'Legal issues in disease outbreaks: judicial review of public health powers', *Health Law Review*, vol 16, no 1, pp 11–16.

Singh, J., Upshur, R. and Padayatchi, N. (2007) 'XDR-TB in South Africa: no time for denial or complacency', *PLoS Medicine*, vol 4, no 1, e50.

Sontag, S. (2001) *Illness as metaphor and AIDS and its metaphors*, New York: Picador.

Upshur, R. (2002) 'Principles for the justification of public health intervention', *Canadian Journal of Public Health*, vol 93, no 2, pp 101–3.

Verma, G., Upshur, R., Rea, E. and Benatar, S. (2004) 'Critical reflections on evidence, ethics and effectiveness in the management of tuberculosis: public health and global perspectives', *BMC Medical Ethics*, vol 5, e2.

WHO (World Health Organization) (2007) *XDR-TB Extensively Drug Resistant Tuberculosis*. Available at: www.who.int/tb/challenges/xdr/en/index.html (accessed 27 August 2008).

FIVE

The evaluation of public health education initiatives on smoking and lung cancer: an ethical critique

Peter Allmark, Angela Tod and Jo Abbott

The focus of this chapter is on ways in which public health information is communicated to the public. In particular it argues that the information concerning the relationship between smoking and lung cancer can convey the wrong messages. The authors' research has shown that the lay public believe that cessation of smoking (or never smoking at all) is almost a guarantee that the individual will not contract lung cancer, and that if this is not the case, they feel in some way 'cheated'. The empirical material demonstrates this very clearly. Their case is that, in order to be more 'ethical', the information given to the public should make it clear that smoking does not inevitably lead to lung cancer and that not smoking cannot guarantee freedom from the disease.

Introduction

This chapter considers the way in which public health education initiatives are evaluated. In particular, our concern is with such evaluation when it is done in terms of behavioural outcomes, such as how many people give up smoking. Our main claim is that this method of evaluation is scientifically and ethically flawed. We use the example of initiatives on smoking and lung cancer. This is because smoking is known to be a hugely important contributor to illness and to health inequality, and because there have been many such initiatives. However, the criticisms we make of initiatives relating to smoking and lung cancer apply equally to many other public health initiatives. Indeed, some criticisms might apply more forcefully to lung cancer initiatives, given that the epidemiological evidence for the link between smoking and lung cancer is stronger than that available for any other link between behaviour and an illness.

We begin the chapter by looking at how health education initiatives in the area of smoking and lung cancer are evaluated. We show that this is done primarily in terms of behaviour change, particularly rates of quitting. We suggest that this is because behaviour change is a good marker for future health benefits which might only accrue over many years: a drop in rates of smoking now could be expected to deliver significant health benefits in the future. However, we argue that looking at behaviour change alone is problematic, because it ignores the possibility of unwanted effects from a public health initiative. We give some evidence for such unwanted effects, based on our own empirical research.

In the light of this we look at two alternative methods of evaluation. The first involves a broader examination of public health initiatives, looking for both desired and undesired effects. This would accord with the usual standard of evidence-based medicine, as in, for example, randomised trials. We argue that while this full-effect evaluation is preferable to evaluation based on behaviour change alone, neither is ethically satisfactory. In particular, it ignores the fact that it would be possible successfully to educate someone about a health issue without that person then deciding to change her behaviour. This is because of the role that people's values play in deciding how to behave. Evaluation that ignores this is compatible with unethical initiatives that, say, deliberately overstate a case in order to achieve the desired health outcome. For this reason, we argue that health education initiatives on lung cancer and smoking should be evaluated primarily as education. On this account, what matters is that health education initiatives provide the information and understanding people need in order to decide whether or not they wish to smoke.

Finally, we consider the issue of whether professionals should target people's values, for example, the values of those who consider smoking a worthwhile pleasure. We argue that it is ethically acceptable in principle, but raises awkward questions concerning which values to target.

What is a public health education initiative?

In the UK at present (2008) the term 'public health education' has a quaint, old-fashioned ring. The government body the Health Education Authority was abolished in 2000 and replaced by the Health Development Authority. The remit of the former included a large role in public education. This disappeared in the remit of the latter, which was to develop the evidence base to improve health and reduce inequality. The Health Development Authority has since been absorbed into the

National Institute for Health and Clinical Excellence (1
is largely concerned with assessing the evidence for the
treatments under the National Health Service (NHS). Whil
of health education has disappeared, 'social marketing' ha.
this bears some resemblance to health education, but we si
that it is significantly different.

We shall need a working definition of public health edu...ation.
Hence: a public health education initiative is one that aims to tackle a
public health problem through education of the public. This chapter
is concerned with such initiatives in the realm of lung cancer and
smoking. An example would be one that aimed to inform smokers
that their habit hugely increases their risk of developing lung cancer.
Such messages are either implicitly or explicitly core elements of
recent education campaigns in the UK. A mix of media has been used,
including television, billboards and newspaper advertisements.

How are public health education initiatives in lung cancer and smoking evaluated?

We have looked at the four key White Papers produced over a 16-year
period that guided service delivery in terms of public health generally,
and more specifically, smoking cessation. Our review began with *The
Health of the Nation* (Department of Health, 1992). This was the first
UK public health policy with measurable targets and outcomes. It
also made clear that health education would be a key component
in government responses to public health problems such as smoking
and lung cancer. The three other White Papers we examined were
Smoking Kills (Department of Health, 1998), *Saving Lives* (Department
of Health, 1999) and *Choosing Health* (Department of Health, 2004).
The first and second of these are located chronologically in the early
years of the New Labour government; the third was published when
New Labour had been in power for seven years. We have analysed
the papers to identify the evaluation or outcome measures set by the
policy in relation to smoking and lung cancer. Our findings are that the
measures of success focus exclusively on behaviour, with no education
outcomes included (Table 5.1). Targets and outcomes relate to reducing
smoking prevalence and cigarette consumption.

This emphasis on behavioural outcomes is seen also in the reviews
of the evidence available regarding smoking and lung cancer. Two
reputable and influential sources of evidence are the Cochrane
Collaboration (www.cochrane.org) and NICE (www.nice.org.uk).
The majority of reviews of evidence on these sites focus on smoking

Table 5.1: Smoking targets from UK health policy 1992–2004

White Paper	Outcome measure
Health of the Nation (1992)	B4/B5: To reduce the death rate for lung cancer by at least 30% in men under 75 and 15% in women under 75 by 2010 (from 60 per 100,000 for men and 24.1 per 100,000 for women in 1990 to no more than 42 and 20.5 respectively). B6/A5: To reduce the prevalence of cigarette smoking in men and women aged 16 and over to no more than 20% by the year 2000 (a reduction of at least 30% in men and 29% in women, from a prevalence in 1990 of 31% and 28% respectively). B7: In addition to reduction in overall prevalence, at least a third of women smokers to stop smoking at the start of their pregnancy by the year 2000. B8: To reduce the consumption of cigarettes by at least 40% by the year 2000 (from 98 billion manufactured cigarettes in 1990 to 59 billion). B9: To reduce smoking prevalence among 11–15-year-olds by at least 33% by 1994 (from about 8% in 1988 to less than 6%).
Saving Lives/ Smoking Kills (1998/1999)	1. To reduce smoking among children from 13% to 9% or less by the year 2010; with a fall to 11% by the year 2005. 2. To reduce adult smoking in all social classes so that the overall rate falls from 28% to 24% or less by the year 2010; with a fall to 26% by the year 2005. 3. To reduce the percentage of women who smoke during pregnancy from 23% to 15% by the year 2010; with a fall to 18% by the year 2005.
Choosing Health (2004)	To reduce adult smoking rates from 26% in 2002 to 21% or less in 2010, with a reduction in prevalence among routine manual groups from 31% in 2002 to 26% or less in 2010.

cessation interventions rather than on education interventions. NICE has published guidance on behaviour change (NICE, 2007). This again indicates an exclusive focus on behaviour over education. It is behaviour change that matters, not what people know about their health.

In response to the *Smoking Kills* White Paper, the government invested heavily in smoking cessation services. Services have employed diverse strategies and activities to address smoking and smoking-related illness. Education is an aspect of some of these approaches; but it is noteworthy that the emphasis on behavioural targets is now reflected in the interventions themselves. For example, in Yorkshire and Humberside a recent (unpublished) document "Achieving four-week quit targets: making it easier for smokers to quit" recommends, inter alia, the following interventions:

- Brief opportunistic advice from a healthcare professional to stop
- Face-to-face intensive behavioural support from a specialist
- Proactive telephone counselling
- Written self-help materials.

In targeting the behaviour of smoking it is clear that smokers are to be put under some pressure to change their life-style.

Why are the initiatives evaluated on the basis of behavioural criteria?

Why are public health education initiatives on lung cancer and smoking primarily evaluated in behavioural terms alone? The answer lies partly in the more general movement towards evidence-based medicine and healthcare. The idea behind this movement is well known and widely accepted. In summary it is as follows: healthcare interventions should be based upon the best available research evidence. All evidence-based healthcare works on the basis of a theory of cause and effect (Harrison, 2003). An action causes an outcome via a mechanism. For example, the action could be giving patients suffering a heart attack a dose of thrombolytic (clot-busting) therapy; the outcome: reducing mortality and morbidity in that group; and the mechanism: the chain of reactions that lead to thrombolysis once the drug is administered. One of the main purposes of healthcare research is to reveal action and outcome and to suggest a mechanism. The focus should be on outcomes that are both measurable and of importance.

In public health the picture is less straightforward. Take our main example: smoking and lung cancer. Here there are two theories in play. The first is the theory of what causes lung cancer: the action is smoking, the outcome is lung cancer and the mechanism is, say, irritation of the mucosa. The evidence base derives from epidemiology. The second theory is of what prevents lung cancer: the action is public health education on smoking and cancer, the outcome is improved public health or reduced levels of lung cancer and the mechanism is people giving up smoking. We make two observations here.

First, with both theories it is difficult to get evidence of the standard of a randomised controlled trial: the public health environment is one in which so many factors are at play that it is hard to control for them all. This is clearly true in epidemiology, which relies on surveying huge numbers to overcome the problem. However, it is also true in the research of public health policy, where a wide range of qualitative and quantitative research is used. The second observation is that it will usually be many years before the desired outcome of the public health education will eventuate. In the light of this, public health professionals concerned with the effectiveness of their interventions will focus evaluation on what can be measured: the mechanism, for example, people quitting smoking. The epidemiological evidence will provide a background that is assumed correct and thus assures the professional that if her action triggers the desired mechanism, the public health benefit will eventually follow.

To summarise: public health education initiatives on lung cancer and smoking are primarily evaluated on behavioural terms alone. This is because the evidence of health benefit from such initiatives is deferred, often by many years. Reference to behavioural change from which health benefit is assumed to flow (on the basis of epidemiological evidence) provides an apparently good alternative; it provides a good fit with evidence-based medicine. For example, epidemiology has established beyond doubt the link between lung cancer and smoking. From this basis professionals can assume that the mechanism, people stopping smoking, will be effective on the outcome, reduced rates of lung cancer. Therefore, they need only assess whether or not their interventions are successful in triggering the mechanism; they know the outcome will follow.

How the initiatives could be evaluated: full effects

One problem with looking at behavioural outcomes alone when evaluating public health initiatives is that it ignores the possibility that there might be other, perhaps harmful, effects that should be set against the benefit of behaviour change. Even in the case of smoking and lung cancer there may be risks or harms as well as benefits from health education initiatives deemed successful in behavioural terms. To illustrate this point we draw on our recent research identifying factors that contribute to a delay in lung cancer diagnosis (Tod et al, 2008). This examined the pathway of people from first symptom to lung cancer diagnosis and identified a number of issues that helped and hindered people in reporting their symptoms to a health professional. The data identified examples of how health education regarding smoking cessation can have unanticipated harmful effects as well as the anticipated benefit of encouraging people to stop smoking. Let us turn to these harmful effects.

First, as with other research (Chapple et al, 2004), the study revealed a prevailing expectation that people with lung cancer would experience blame and stigma. Participants reported an expectation that smokers would be blamed and held responsible for developing lung cancer. This belief was reinforced by the tone of 'stop smoking' education campaigns and the way in which health professionals had treated smokers in the past.

> Whenever you see warnings about cancer, there's always a cigarette there. I don't think I've seen a warning where there hasn't been a cigarette and I think that's wrong. (68-year-old male with terminal lung cancer, ex-smoker of 25 years)

> I've got a friend who has a hacking cough because she smokes and I'm always saying to her, "you ought to get that looked at." She said, "I'm not going to the doctor because the minute they find out I'm a smoker I get in trouble". So you don't go because you don't want to be ticked off. (Wife of 67-year-old male with terminal lung cancer, ex-smoker of 25 years)

There was a perception that smokers would be stigmatised and seen as undeserving of healthcare. This perception created a sense of being ostracised and added to delay in symptom reporting.

> I mean it's all been focused on smoking and I'm not denying that that is what probably caused my cancer and other people's cancer, but, ... I don't know, by dictatorial ways or pressing people, making you feel ostracised, doesn't work! (65-year-old woman, 18-month survivor of lung cancer following lung resection, ex-smoker who gave up on diagnosis)

Interestingly, even those who were non- or ex-smokers delayed in reporting symptoms because of an expectation that they would be stigmatised as smokers and blamed for their illness. This expectation was reinforced by experience. Health professionals assumed that they were smokers and kept asking about smoking status.

> They keep asking have I smoked? Have I drunk? It's mainly have I smoked ... anytime? I say, "No." The only thing I have is gone into bingo where there's been smoke. (63-year-old woman with terminal lung cancer, non-smoker)

Thus the tone and content of smoking-cessation health education campaigns may promote delay in symptom reporting, contributing to delayed diagnosis and a poorer chance of survival.

Second, in health education campaigns lung cancer is used as a threat to promote smoking cessation. On the basis of such education campaigns some ex-smokers and non-smokers believed they were not at risk of lung cancer. The following scenario illustrates the point. Two men had both given up smoking over 20 years ago, each on the birth of his first child. This was motivated by a desire to protect the health of the child and to be healthy and provide for the child's future. The decision was influenced by a belief, derived from health education messages, that if they gave up smoking their lungs would be clear and their risk of lung cancer would be nil.

> I packed up smoking and then after ten years you hear stories, you know, "well, it's all cleared out your system and everything" and I thought, I'm never going to get lung cancer or any other one come to that. I'm not smoking. (68-year-old male with terminal lung cancer, ex-smoker of 25 years)

This belief that they were not at risk of lung cancer meant that, as symptoms emerged and got worse, they continued to ignore them or to explain them away as something else.

> I mean I gave up 25 years ago so you almost forgot that you ever were a smoker. (67-year-old male with terminal lung cancer, ex-smoker of 25 years)

> If he'd been a smoker and he was getting breathless and he ... his irritating cough had got worse it would be different.... we might well have said, "Hang on, you'd better get this looked at". I think everybody associates lung cancer with smoking and if you don't smoke they assume you're not at risk. (Wife)

An additional issue to emerge from the experiences of these two participants was the lack of awareness of the risks of second-hand smoke. Both men thought their risk of lung cancer was nil after stopping smoking. This was despite working and socialising in smoky atmospheres. It was only after diagnosis that they realised the lung cancer risk from passive smoking.

> But he worked in a smoky atmosphere and … I think most people think, "Oh, I don't smoke. I'm safe," and that's not true … But the message that comes across is that it's the cancer of the smoker, so if you're not a smoker you can sit back and think, "Well, I'm not going to get that". (Wife of 67-year-old male with terminal lung cancer, ex-smoker of 25 years)

Thus, public health education initiatives can have negative consequences even where the epidemiological evidence is exceptionally strong, as it is with lung cancer and smoking. This gives us our case for a fuller assessment of health education initiatives – not just in terms of whether they work on behaviour change or not, but in terms of whether they have other, unanticipated effects. In other words, such initiatives should be judged as other health initiatives are judged, on all of their effects, and not simply on their desirable ones.

Someone defending the behavioural method of evaluation might respond that any ill effects of successful education initiatives to reduce smoking will easily be outweighed by the benefits; spending time and money measuring the ill effects would be pointless. To deploy such an argument, the evidence would need to assure a very strong health benefit from a public health mechanism. It is arguable that this is the case with smoking and lung cancer. Even then, however, failing to look for the negative aspects of health education initiatives seems to block the way to improving future initiatives. On these grounds alone we believe the full-effects evaluation is superior to the behaviour-based evaluation.

There is one further, speculative point that might add support for using the full-effects evaluation rather than behaviour evaluation. Public health agencies are charged with reducing health inequality. But the adverse outcomes of health education initiatives might be such as to fall disproportionately in deprived areas, and thus increase inequality. The adverse effects certainly occur in areas of deprivation (Tod and Craven, 2006; Tod et al, 2008). They also occur disproportionately: South Yorkshire is a relatively deprived area which suffers rates of lung cancer much higher than the national average; and within South Yorkshire, the most deprived areas have the highest lung cancer rates (Directors of Public Health of South Yorkshire, 2006). In that health inequality is itself a problem that needs addressing, the full-effects evaluation should be undertaken. It could be, for example, that misunderstanding of public health information is greater in areas of deprivation. If that were so, then such information could contribute to increases in inequality.

Overall, therefore, we believe that it is better for those involved in health education to evaluate the possible unexpected and ill effects of their initiatives, not simply to assume on the basis of epidemiology that behaviour change will lead to overwhelming benefit. This is of import also to social marketing, the application of marketing methods that are usually used to effect consumer behaviour change, to effect population health behaviour change (Grier and Bryant, 2005). Its sole focus on behaviour change makes it vulnerable to our criticism of the behavioural method of evaluation.

How the initiatives could be evaluated: education and attitudes

However, even full-effects evaluation of public health education initiatives in the area of lung cancer and smoking is problematic. There is a conceptual difference between health education and health treatment. A health treatment has the unproblematic goal (usually) of improving health in some way. With education, the goal is usually to educate: that people will gain knowledge or skills. Public health education could be evaluated in such a way: for example, we could evaluate initiatives on the basis of whether or not people learnt the relevant facts about smoking, lung cancer and health.

This conceptual difference marks a significant ethical difference (Buchanan, 2006). In the previous section we showed a number of people who either gave up smoking or never smoked, at least in part because of health education initiatives. If we were to ask whether these initiatives were successful on the basis of behaviour change, then clearly they were: people gave up smoking. Similarly, on the basis of overall effects, the initiatives were successful: although some of the cancer sufferers had a delayed diagnosis because of false beliefs gained through health education, they nonetheless benefited overall; had they continued to smoke they would very likely have died much sooner. However, if we were to evaluate the initiatives in terms of health education, our response would be different: these people had not learnt all the relevant facts about smoking; indeed, they had taken on some false beliefs. It was not a success.

Of course, there may not necessarily be a conflict between the full-effects and education approaches. It may be that the health benefits would have been even greater if people had taken on true beliefs at the outset: for example, knowing that ceasing smoking hugely reduces but does not eliminate the risk of lung cancer. But there is a genuine tension here. Should health education be viewed as propaganda for health in which overstated or even deceitful claims can be made? Would it matter were people to believe smoking to be more dangerous than it is, and stopping smoking more beneficial, so long as they gave up?

These questions mirror a classic stand-off between utilitarian and non-utilitarian ethical positions, the former defending deception, the latter decrying it (Jackson, 2001; Kozlowski and Edwards, 2005). Perhaps it is unlikely that many would defend deception of the population in order to effect behaviour change. Nonetheless, the evaluation of health education using either the behavioural method or the (better) full-effects analysis invites the view that the good obtained through changing smoking behaviour outweighs any concerns about, for example, over-advocacy. By contrast, from other viewpoints it is important that we convey information in such a way that people are able to weigh up true information and make decisions on that basis, even if those decisions are not what we want them to be. It is difficult to give an overwhelming argument against the utilitarian defence of deception or over-advocacy. However, we do not generally accept anything less than informed consent to treatment in other areas of healthcare; it is unclear why health education should be different.

There is an alternative, non-utilitarian defence of using full-effects rather than the health education criteria. Someone might say that there is no need for deception; the facts are clear enough. Once people fully understand the dangers of smoking, then almost all will want to give up or not start. The only additional point healthcare professionals should bear in mind is the need to help people overcome addiction or peer pressure. For reasons that will become apparent, we call this the shared-values argument. It is an argument that appears to underlie much public health policy. For example, in the White Paper *Choosing Health* (discussed earlier) there is frequent slippage between the terms "healthy choice" and "informed choice". The implication is that no properly informed person would make an unhealthy choice. Let us set out this argument in more detail before going on to show its problems.

Discussing this argument requires first that we set out a basic model of human action. Because public health professionals have been concerned with people's health behaviour they have been interested in action theory: theory concerned with why people act as they do. Such theory belongs primarily to the realms of psychology and philosophy. Various models have been employed (Azjen, 1991; Megone, 2000; Tones and Tilford, 2001; Allmark, 2005). From these it is possible to identify a simple action theory that will suffice for our discussion here. This can be written formulaically in the following way:

$$\text{factual beliefs} + \text{values} + \text{perceived behaviour control} =$$
$$\text{intention} \approx \text{action}$$

The component 'factual beliefs' is straightforward here; we mean those beliefs that you have about the world that you believe to be true. You might, of course, be in error. Your values are your beliefs about things that are worth having or avoiding in life – philosophers sometimes call this your vision of the good. Perceived behaviour control is your belief about whether you are able to perform the action or not. So, if someone believes smoking is linked to lung cancer, highly values his health and believes he can give up, then he is likely to form the intention to give up. He will not necessarily go from intention to action: for example, because of addiction.

From the shared values perspective, values remain constant across different people – we all place a high value on good health. Therefore, people's smoking behaviour is viewed as depending on their factual beliefs and their perceived behaviour control. The thought then is that, aside from public health education aimed at informing people of the risks, the other need is for public health measures aimed at, say, reducing peer pressure (such as limiting areas of smoking) and overcoming addiction (for example, providing nicotine substitutes).

The fault in the shared-values picture lies in the assumption that we all value good health similarly. That this is not true is shown by the risky behaviour that some people indulge in, where their perceived behaviour control is likely to be high (for example, climbing). What the shared-values picture misses is the chance that people will see positive aspects to smoking. Hilary Graham's research suggests something to this effect (Graham, 1987). Young unmarried mothers in deprived areas to whom she spoke valued the present benefits of smoking, for example, in giving them time to themselves, more highliy than they disvalued future harms. The shared-values argument also misses the possibility that some people may not particularly value a long life – if cigarettes provide solace in a fairly unhappy life, then there seems to be little reason to give up. Smoking may be part of a subculture in which rebelliousness against authority is valued (Ling and Glantz, 2002). Hence, there can be a pro-attitude to smoking. It follows that the shared-values argument is wrong: people could have the same factual beliefs about smoking and about behaviour control, but have different values. Hence the shared-values argument cannot be used as a non–utilitarian defence of using the full-effects criterion in evaluating public health education initiatives.[1]

To sum up: we have argued that the full–effects evaluation of public health education is preferable to evaluating only behaviour change. However, both methods are vulnerable to the criticism that they are compatible with the use of deception and propagandising. We have examined two responses to this criticism. The first is that deception is justified for the good cause of the nation's health. We argued that this is probably not compatible with an ethos of informed consent and respect for autonomy. The second is that deception is not necessary: accurately informed people will make the right choices. We only need to assess the extent to which people make the right choices in order to know whether or not they are properly informed. We showed that this argument depends on a shared-values view. We argued that while this view seems to be reflected in public health literature, it is problematic.

By default, this leaves us with the education approach to evaluation of public health education initiatives. If healthcare professionals were to take this approach to evaluation, then it would be ethically acceptable for them to engage with people's factual beliefs and with their perceived behaviour control. Hence, if people don't believe smoking is harmful, or believe their addiction is insurmountable, public health education initiatives could correct these beliefs. However, a critic of this approach might say that it does nothing to address pro-attitude smokers, those who currently see smoking as positive overall. This is unlike the full-effects and behaviour approaches, where one is entitled to tackle smoking in whatever way is necessary.

How might a defender of the education method of evaluation respond? It is true that at the heart of the education approach is the ethical idea that it is wrong deliberately to distort or frame information in order to get a desired behavioural outcome. This is a matter of principle, something like the principle of respect for autonomy. To some extent it is also a matter of practicality. Health education initiatives lose credibility if they are based on distortion; this is reflected in the emergence of an alternative 'lay epidemiology' (Davison, Smith and Frankel, 1991; Frankel, Davison and Smith, 1991; Allmark and Tod, 2006). However, it does not follow that public health initiatives should not target people's values. From the perspective of the education approach there is no reason, in principle, not to. The ethical case for or against doing so will come down to wider ethical beliefs.

The case against engaging with people's values might begin from an assumption that it is wrong to impose your values on others. As an example, it might be argued that it is wrong to make abortion illegal, as this imposes anti-abortion views on those who don't share them. In the context of health education, the argument might be that it is wrong to try to change people's minds about what is and is not of value in their lives. If someone has a pro-attitude to smoking despite knowing the medical facts, then health education should leave it at that. Such a view will tend to draw on the idea that values are outside of rational criticism. For example, some people like cakes or smoking, others do not; there are no rational arguments that would persuade individuals to change their values.

However, this position can be challenged. There appear to be some values that we do believe to be wrong; for example, torturing for fun. In that we hold this to be wrong we are generally able to give reasons or arguments to defend our view. This would suggest that values are amenable to argument. On this account, someone who believes that the pleasure of smoking now outweighs the future harm might be mistaken. It would therefore be reasonable to engage with that person with a view to helping her see aright.

Holding that people can be mistaken in their values does not require that you believe that the same values should hold for all people. A full discussion of the rights and wrongs of smoking for an individual might still result in that person retaining a pro-attitude to smoking. On the other hand, that individual might come to believe that he has not sufficiently evaluated, say, the effect of his early death on those around him. As a result, his pro-attitude may change. This argument could be reinforced by reference to certain basic shared values, such as good health. Although it is not the case that we all value health equally, because some of us are willing to risk it or even lose it for other goods, it is certainly the case that for almost all people it is better not to be ill, other things being equal.

We suggest, then, that public health professionals could be justified in tackling people's values, helping them think about whether they have got them right. Public health professionals probably do this already under descriptions such as 'changing attitudes' or 'changing cultures' (as in tackling the culture of binge drinking in the UK). A good example is a television advertisement in which a young girl spoke to an interviewer about her father who was dying of lung cancer. She spoke very movingly about him and what she thought of smoking. This advert was not really concerned with conveying information; it was asking smokers to rethink their attitude to the habit, to re-evaluate.

So it is not necessarily objectionable in principle for professionals to engage with people's values, with a view to changing them. There is, however, a difficult problem here. Why should we focus on those with a pro-attitude to smoking rather than on those with a pro-attitude to other risky behaviour, such as climbing, horse-riding or driving? Why are there no adverts asking climbers and horse-riders to think about taking up a safer sport; or drivers to travel less and use lower-risk transportation?

The answer is perhaps that smoking combines a unique set of factors: it risks harm to others; it is unpleasant to many; there is an element of addiction among those with the pro-attitude; it is a major cause of avoidable harm; the epidemiological evidence is strong; and both the habit and the pro-attitude are probably concentrated in relatively poor and powerless groups, while its disparagers are wealthier and more powerful. If this answer is along the right lines, then the justification for intervention is clearly not straightforward. It follows that it is not straightforward to say which health values professionals should tackle. It seems revealing that many public health campaigns are focused on areas that encompass traditional vices: intemperance (smoking and drinking); gluttony (obesity); sloth (exercise); and lust (sexual health). Perhaps this underlines Buchanan's (2006) point, that health education is a moral and political enterprise. If so, public health professionals tread a line between justified advice and unjustified moralising.

Conclusion

Using the example of smoking and lung cancer, we have argued that public health education initiatives should not be evaluated solely on the basis of behavioural outcomes or overall (full-effects) outcomes. The latter is better than the former, in that it involves looking for undesired side effects of your interventions as well as determining whether they had the desired effect of changing behaviour. However, both fall foul of a non-utilitarian ethic that disallows deception. If only behaviour change or health outcomes matter, then the way we achieve those outcomes is of less concern; if deception is necessary to change behaviour, then perhaps it should be deployed. We argued that this is not the spirit in which health education should be conducted; that is, as a medium for imparting knowledge. We also argued that it might be appropriate to use health education as a focus for personal reflection on values. There is little ethical problem in justifying health education initiatives on lung cancer and smoking, because the epidemiological evidence is so strong. However, the case for initiatives that tackle values is more complex and subtle. Health is almost universally of value to people; knowing that some activities pose immense risk to health helps them in making decisions. But public health professionals perhaps need to take stock before embarking on value-based campaigns, such as the tearful girl. They should ask: why the pro-attitude smokers; why the culture of binge drinking; why teenage sex; and why not teenage horse riding, middle-aged drivers and exercise addicts with crumbling joints? Insofar as health education initiatives seek to change people's values as well as their knowledge, professionals need to think carefully about whether and why they are justified in doing so.

Acknowledgement
We wish to thank the anonymous referee for extensive comments on an earlier draft.

Note
[1] The existence of pro-attitude smokers would raise a problem for those charged with meeting ever-rising targets of smokers quitting. The likelihood is that early campaigns will meet with success, as those who want to give up are helped to do so. Far more difficult will be the remainder, who have no desire to quit.

References

Allmark, P. (2005) 'Health, happiness and health promotion', *Journal of Applied Philosophy*, vol 22, no 1, pp 1–15.

Allmark, P. and Tod, A. (2006) 'How should public health professionals engage with lay epidemiology?' *Journal of Medical Ethics*, vol 32, no 8, pp 460–3.

Azjen, I. (1991) 'The theory of planned behaviour', *Organizational Behavior and Human Decision Processes*, vol 50, no 2, pp 179–212.

Buchanan, D. (2006) 'Perspective: A new ethic for health promotion: Reflections on a philosophy of health education for the 21st century', *Health Education & Behavior*, vol 33, no 3, pp 290–304.

Chapple, A., Ziebland, S. and McPherson, A. (2004) 'Stigma, shame, and blame experienced by patients with lung cancer: Qualitative study', *British Medical Journal*, vol 328, no 7454, p 1470.

Davison, C., Smith, G.D. and Frankel, S. (1991) 'Lay epidemiology and the prevention paradox – the implications of coronary candidacy for health-education', *Sociology of Health & Illness*, vol 13, no 1, pp 1–19.

Department of Health (1992) *The health of the nation*, London: HMSO.

Department of Health (1998) *Smoking kills*, London: HMSO.

Department of Health (1999) *Saving lives: Our healthier nation*, London: HMSO.

Department of Health (2004) *Choosing health: Making health choices easier*, London: HMSO.

Directors of Public Health of South Yorkshire (2006) *Improving health: Narrowing the divide*. Available at: www.doncasterpct.nhs.uk/documents/introduction.pdf (accessed 6 February 2009).

Frankel, S., Davison, C. and Smith, G.D. (1991) 'Lay epidemiology and the rationality of responses to health- education', *British Journal of General Practice*, vol 41, no 351, pp 428–30.

Graham, H. (1987) 'Women's smoking and family health', *Social Science & Medicine*, vol 25, no 1, pp 47–56.

Grier, S. and Bryant, C. (2005) 'Social marketing in public health', *Annual Review of Public Health*, vol 26, pp 319–39.

Harrison, T. (2003) 'Evidence-based multidisciplinary public health', in J. Orme, J. Powell, P. Taylor and M. Grey (eds) *Public health for the 21st century*, Maidenhead: Open University Press, pp 227–45.

Jackson, J. (2001) *Truth, trust and medicine*, London: Routledge.

Kozlowski, L. and Edwards, B. (2005) '"Not safe" is not enough: Smokers have a right to know more than there is no safe tobacco product', *Tobacco Control*, vol 14, Suppl 2, pp 3–7.

Ling, P. and Glantz, S. (2002) 'Using tobacco-industry marketing research to design more effective tobacco-control campaigns', *Journal of the American Medical Association*, vol 287, no 22, pp 2983–9.

Megone, C. (2000) 'Potentiality and persons: An Aristotelian perspective', in M. Kuczewski and R. Polansky (eds) *Bioethics*, London: MIT Press, pp 155–78.

NICE (2007) *Behaviour change at population, community and individual levels*, London: NICE.

Tod, A. and Craven, J. (2006) *Diagnostic delay in lung cancer: Barriers and facilitators in diagnostic delay*, Sheffield: University of Sheffield.

Tod, A., Craven, J. and Allmark, P. (2008) 'Diagnostic delay in lung cancer: A qualitative study', *Journal of Advanced Nursing*, vol 61, no 3, pp 336–43.

Tones, K. and Tilford, S. (2001) *Health promotion: Effectiveness, efficiency and equity*, Cheltenham: Nelson Thornes.

SIX

Relevance of primary care bioethics committees in public health ethical practice in the community: an experience in an area of extreme poverty in Santiago, Chile

Marla Solari and Tatiana Escobar-Koch

Public health ethics is highly context sensitive, and the ethical judgements that are made depend on the culture concerned. This chapter is concerned with the very real difficulties encountered in dealing with ethical problems that arise in a community setting, and is a broadly descriptive account of how dilemmas are resolved through a family healthcare bioethics committee in Chile. It contains some detailed accounts of case studies which illustrate how, in a very real sense, ethical ideas have to be translated into practice.

Introduction

Bioethics is perceived as applied ethics, in other words, the place of interaction between ethical concern and a specific sphere of practice characterised by the prefix 'bio' (Ladrière, 2000). Thus, bioethics applies to dilemmas of value which arise in particular spheres of action in relation to the phenomenon of life, its manifestations and interactions. However, bioethics has not been sufficiently explored from the perspective of primary healthcare, where significant ethical conflicts and dilemmas occur. The variety and complexity of ethical dilemmas in primary healthcare derive from the continuous, bio-psychosocial interaction of the healthcare teams and the community, and they imply particular responsibilities of the state and of society as a whole.

Primary healthcare is the principal pathway to health services in public health systems and it interacts daily with individuals, families and communities. It is, to a great extent, the area in charge of promoting healthy life-styles, preventing illness and recovering the health of individuals (Zurro and Pérez, 2000). The role of primary healthcare became evident in the World Health Organization's (WHO) international primary healthcare conference at Alma-Ata in 1978. At that meeting it was once more reiterated not only that health is the absence of disease, but that it encompasses the overall state of physical, psychological and social well-being of the individual, family and society (WHO, 1978). It implies promoting health through healthy life-styles, preventing diseases and accidents, maintaining people with chronic diseases, and rehabilitating their health when necessary. It is evident that this requires the collaboration and coordination of different sectors. Among them, primary healthcare has a relevant role, due to the closeness of its healthcare teams to the community, its institutions and organisations, its families and their life-styles, and to the continuous care provided by primary healthcare to each individuals throughout their life-cycle. This becomes most apparent in a family healthcare model (MINSAL, 1999a).

During the primary healthcare conference at Alma-Ata, there was also a consensus that health is a fundamental human right and that achieving a healthy population is an important social objective (WHO, 1978). This is why governments, healthcare personnel and the worldwide community insist on strengthening and reorienting healthcare systems,

Figure 6.1: The Cristo Vive Primary Care Family Health Centre

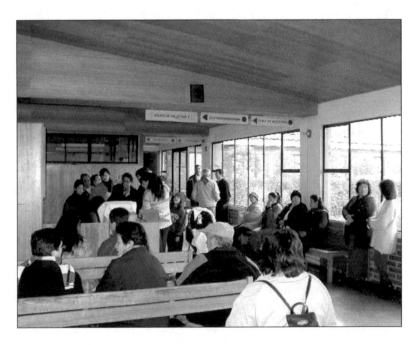

emphasising the relevant role primary healthcare fulfils towards meeting that objective (WHO, 1978). It is therefore unlikely that there could be another area with a greater need of critical ethical reflection regarding its actions than primary healthcare and its complex network of urban and rural clinics, primary healthcare emergency services or attached clinics, and family healthcare centres, as they occur in Chile and in many other countries (Solari, 2003).

Because of the context in which primary healthcare develops, it is not surprising that the ethical dilemmas that arise involve different sectors of the community and that social, family and couple conflicts become evident (Gracia, 1989). Likewise, the political, economic and cultural situations of a country become evident through the diversity of the individual communities served by the primary healthcare teams. Thus, primary healthcare is in a privileged position and has a concrete possibility of protecting the varied and particular interests of human life in our communities in a responsible and systematic way.

Ethics is the branch of philosophy dedicated to critical reflection with regard to the fundamentals of individual and collective human acts, whether they are classified as good or bad (Thompson, 2000), which implies a general view about the purpose and nature of human life. However, we know that at present a significant proportion of the world population are living in conditions that can be classified as inhuman (Velasco, 1996) and that there are critical situations which can even endanger human survival on the planet, such as severe social and cultural conflicts. Thus, by identifying and analysing bioethical dilemmas in specific spheres of community life – or in the primary healthcare team, which is close to their reality – it may be possible to seek solutions to the eventual ethical contradictions that may arise in those contexts, and to take concrete steps to forestall problems that emerge and that have implications for the health and well-being of the community. Furthermore, from a broader and more ambitious perspective, this may contribute towards protecting the life of future generations.

The practice of bioethics is based on knowledge, experience and rules in a particular context. Therefore it is expected that, on the basis of particular experiences, we may infer elements that may make it possible to judge or guide ethical practice, establish rules and, based on what they suggest (inductive method), acquire greater knowledge. This method has been the basis of the development of bioethics, a casuistic discussion and a model that permits the establishment of proposals, criteria and even general principles (Ladrière, 2000).

This chapter examines a specific primary healthcare experience, that of the Cristo Vive family healthcare centre and its bioethics committee. Examples of cases that are brought before the bioethics committee are provided and two cases are examined in detail to demonstrate the way in which the committee works. The analysis was approached using the methodology proposed by Gracia (1989). On the basis of these cases, we shall see whether it is possible to infer elements that enable us to guide bioethical practice. The idea is to make contributions based on a particular, local or regional bioethical analysis by discovering its peculiarities (Rosselot, 1998; Ladrière, 2000). Before examining the cases that characterise an area of bioethics for primary healthcare, some background information about the Chilean context is provided.

Bioethics: the Chilean context

Bioethics emerges within the conflicts of value regarding life that are generated in developed societies as a result of techno-scientific development. Further development occurs within the frame of that particular culture and vision of the world. Although Latin American countries have to face the same value conflicts as the developed world, other bioethical problems arise from deficient social conditions that affect vulnerable groups. A significant proportion of Latin American people are economically deprived. In 2005, 39.8% of the Latin American population lived in poverty, defined as having an income amounting to less than twice the cost of a basic food basket (ECLAC, 2007). Of these, 10.3% lived in conditions of indigence, with incomes amounting to less than the cost of one basic food basket (ECLAC, 2007).

In Chile, due to significant economic development, the percentage of people living in poverty has decreased substantially over the last decades. In 1990, 25.6% of the population were poor (but not indigent) and 13% were indigent, whereas by 2006 these numbers had dropped to 10.5% (poor but not indigent) and 3.2% (indigent) (MIDEPLAN, 2006). Despite these advances, important inequities still exist and people living in poverty have higher illiteracy and unemployment rates, and fewer than average years of schooling (MIDEPLAN, 2006). Moreover, if a broader definition of poverty is considered, which includes not only lack of adequate food, clean water, sanitation services, proper housing, and access to education and healthcare, but also lack of quality interpersonal relations, loneliness and lack of face-to-face encounters with others (United Nations, 1992), it becomes even clearer that the marginalisation and harsh disadvantages faced by underprivileged sectors of the community generate important bioethical dilemmas.

Ethnic minorities constitute another vulnerable segment of the population in Latin America, and in Chile the nine indigenous ethnic groups recognised by the state account for 6.6% of the population (MIDEPLAN, 2006). Although in the last few years the gap between the indigenous and the non-indigenous population has narrowed considerably, indigenous groups continue to have higher levels of poverty and indigence, as well as higher illiteracy rates, fewer average years of schooling, and lower average salaries than the non-indigenous population (MIDEPLAN, 2006). In addition, important cultural differences exist and have the potential to cause tensions between diverse communities. In these situations, bioethics committees may act as intercultural mediators seeking consensus through dialogue and debate – what is known as intercultural bioethics.

In addition to addressing dilemmas faced by vulnerable sectors of the population, the role of community bioethics becomes increasingly important in the face of profound social and cultural changes which have taken place in the community, such as changes in the structure of the family, in gender roles, in values regarding sexuality and in religious identification, among others (Méndez, 2002). They create various ethical dilemmas between health teams, service users and the community, often complicating health decisions (Rosselot, 1998). The bioethics committee and its methodology, which generates discussion and facilitates consensus, thus sets the stage for the elaboration and implementation of community health policies on issues such as responsible sexuality, family violence and the community life of people with HIV and other chronic illnesses.

Chile, the capital of which is Santiago, is located on the south-western coast of South America. It is 4,270 kilometres in length and has great topographic diversity. It has a democratic government and a population of just under 15.12 million (Instituto Nacional de Estadísticas, 2002). The Chilean health system is divided into two sub-systems, one public and one private. Technically, both are ruled and regulated by the Ministry of Health.

The public health system serves over 70% of the population (71.6% in 2003), including the poorest people in the country (MINSAL, 2006). Its services are provided through the National Health Services system, with 28 autonomous services throughout the country and a very well-organised network of primary care health centres, specialist technological clinics and hospitals. It includes the National Health Fund (FONASA), the Institute of Public Health, the National Supply Centre and the Metropolitan Environmental Health Service.

The private health system is constituted of people or institutions that, with or without economic interest, provide health services such as medical centres, health clinics, hospitals, laboratories, pharmacies and so on. They do not have to execute Ministry of Health programmes but are nonetheless governed by the state sanitary code. They are not part of a formal network and offer their services in the free market. Most people who access healthcare in this system belong to the private insurance system (ISAPRES) (16.7% of the population in 2003), which is supervised by the Superintendent of ISAPRES (MINSAL, 2006). There is an additional autonomous health system for the armed forces and police force.

The Cristo Vive primary care family health centre

The biomedical model still dominates the health sector in Chile, with great interest in specialised technology and hospitals. However, in recent decades health reform has been taking place that emphasises primary healthcare and the family bio-psychosocial model, although it has met with some resistance. The Cristo Vive primary care family health centre is a pilot for the model in Chile. Indeed, the community bioethics reflection developed from its history and mission. The Cristo Vive family health centre is part of the Cristo Vive Foundation, a private, non-profit organisation founded and directed by Sister Karoline Mayer Hofbeck. It is based on a Christian mission and has a history of advocating for human rights (Fundación Cristo Vive, 2000).

The centre serves, free of charge, 20,000 people from a very deprived area of north Santiago. It is part of the public health system network and receives financial support from FONASA, follows all the Ministry of Health's programmes and is evaluated by it. However, it is managed by the Cristo Vive Foundation, whose interest is the Christian mission of the institution. It thus represents a new private–public collaboration within the country. It is also a university centre, with over 500 students from different health professions doing practical rotations throughout the year.

The centre has implemented a family bio–psychosocial primary care model. Structurally, service users are assigned to one of four sectors, each with a basic family care team in charge: a family doctor, nurse, midwife, technician and secretary. In addition, different professionals complement their work, for example nutritionists, health social workers, psychologists, dentists and kinesiologists. The entire range of individual and family needs is covered, with various programmes oriented towards promoting health and preventing illness, in coordination with the community. The main health problems of the population are linked with psychosocial problems and include drug addiction, alcoholism,

Figure 6.2: The Cristo Vive Bioethics Committee at work

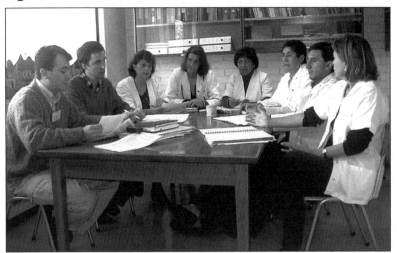

family violence, teenage pregnancy, and prostitution, as well as chronic illnesses, accidents and others.

The bioethics committee

As has been established, bioethics is essential in primary care public health centres, due to the conflicts of value that arise in the interaction of the primary healthcare teams with the community and the public health network. The bioethics discipline uses a committee methodology to analyse and solve ethical dilemmas. It is based on an open, systematic and plural dialogue between people coming from different disciplines, belief systems and worldviews (Beca and Kottow, 1996). This 'bioethics committee methodology' allows a consensus to be reached, which is especially valued in poor and intercultural communities such as Villa Los Heroes ex Angela Davis, the underprivileged area of Santiago where the Cristo Vive family health centre is located.

The motivation for using this methodology stemmed from a combination of four factors:

- from Frau Karoline Mayer and her mission;
- from the context in which the Foundation developed, a low-income community with a history of advocating for the defence of human rights;
- from the participation of one of the authors of this chapter, who holds a Masters degree in Bioethics;
- from a very motivated team.

The committee has gone through three stages of development. The first was group formation and cohesion. The Cristo Vive bioethics committee began operating in 1999. At this stage objectives and roles were defined and the work methodology was established. The second stage was experiential, where cases were presented to facilitate discussion of issues relevant to primary healthcare, such as informed consent, confidentiality, birth-rate regulation and contraceptive methods, the day-after pill and patients' rights. In the third stage the committee went through a consolidation phase, characterised by the systematic analysis of dilemmas that arise in relation to healthcare and have bioethical repercussions.

The objectives of the committee are to recognise cases distinctive for primary healthcare and, in the longer term, to analyse, deliberate, reach a consensus and formulate recommendations in relation to cases and bioethical quandaries that arise from the praxis of the primary healthcare team. The committee also prepares guidance and institutional ethics policies in relation to routine work and special programmes in primary healthcare, and offers continuous training and education to its members, the healthcare team and the community. The committee has eight permanent members: two doctors, one nurse, one priest, one lawyer, one member of the community, one psychologist and one occupational therapist. In some sessions there is also an occasional attendee. The competency selection process considered interest in and knowledge of bioethics. Three members have Masters degrees in Bioethics and two have Bioethics diplomas. All levels of the organisation are represented on the committee, including the community.

When a service user, member of the healthcare team or other professional has an ethical dilemma, the case is presented to the committee president, who determines whether it is pertinent. If the case is not appropriate, the person is directed to the appropriate body. If it is pertinent, a date is set for a 20-minute presentation of the family's clinical and socio-economic background and the ethical dilemma. The presentation is made before the bioethics committee, which meets monthly for an hour and a half. The members of the committee then deliberate and debate the case. This includes discussion of all the alternatives, ethical principles which are compromised and the best interests of those involved. When a consensus is reached, the committee formulates its recommendations, which are communicated in writing. Follow-up of the case must then be made, and news reports are discussed at subsequent meetings. Examples of ethical dilemmas that have been presented to the committee are illustrated in Table 6.1.

Table 6.1: Examples of ethical dilemmas affecting service users or the primary healthcare team

Example	Reason brought to the committee
Unit: Family health centre *Presented by:* Family healthcare team social worker *Case:* Inquiry made by 56-year-old widow regarding her 5-year-old grandchild who attends the Cristo Vive Foundation kindergarten. The grandmother suspects that the child's father is sexually abusing him. The child's mother denies this, despite some physical injuries presented by the child which seem to support the accusations of abuse, but which cannot be confirmed at the Medical Legal Institute, due to the mother's refusal. The family is afraid of the father.	The health team requests support to determine how to act in the child's best interest. Who represents the child's best interest: the grandmother, the mother, or the health team? What is the degree of autonomy of the family in relation to the health team? Can the team intervene? Is the involvement of the health team beneficent or maleficent in this case?
Unit: Family health centre *Presented by:* Family doctor *Case:* Four siblings aged 7 years and under at bio-psychosocial risk. This is a family of high biological, psychological and social risk that does not attend appointments at the health centre for vaccinations or family planning, and the children's school attendance is poor. There is a possibility of a new (unwanted) pregnancy and the family depends on the income from the father's sporadic jobs. The oldest daughter is interned in a state home, and the home's team feels the rest of the siblings should be placed there. The Cristo Vive health team has repeatedly attempted to change the attitude of the family, but this has generated anger on its part and withdrawal from the health centre, and has gone so far as threats to the health professionals. The health team feels both alternatives for the children (state home or remaining in their own home) are potentially harmful.	Is it the health team's duty to intervene and protect the girls? Is it above the family's autonomy? What are the rights of negligent parents? Is the common welfare the limit to the autonomy of this family? Who is responsible for this family: the state, the town council, the local health council? Is there paternalism on the part of the health team? Does the family prioritise its needs differently from the health team? Who best represents the girls' best interest?

continued

91

Table 6.1: *continued*

Example	Reason brought to the committee
Unit: Administration *Presented by:* Health team *Case:* Policy of the health centre regarding hiring personnel and accepting volunteers gives priority to people of the village, to which the majority of the patients belong. The people are integrated into the health teams and have access to confidential information about patients, often their own neighbours or even family.	Is it a maleficent or beneficent policy to hire personnel from the same community, knowing that they have access to confidential information, but that at the same time they best take care of the health centre and also represent the interests of the community?
Unit: Administration *Presented by:* Director *Case:* A study (double blind, randomised, placebo-controlled study for treatment of children with influenza) has contemplated a payment of US$50 to each professional who detects a case and an additional US$50 for the health centre.	Is this payment ethical?
Unit: Family health centre *Presented by:* Family healthcare team *Case:* Chronically ill patient who suffers from morbid obesity, hypertension and diabetes. Patient does not come for health checks or comply with treatment. The professionals follow the Ministry of Health technical guidance, repeatedly explaining the risks to the patient, but patient does not respond.	Which has precedence, the patient's autonomy or the health team's recommendations? Must the health team impose its guidance on this patient?

Committee achievements and challenges

Over time, the objectives, roles and methods of working of the bioethics committee have changed, improving their approach. In particular, local health workers are more aware of the importance and identification of bioethical issues, which in turn supports the work of the committee. Thus, the importance of the bioethics committee and its contribution towards enriching the family primary healthcare model are recognised by the primary healthcare team and local public health network. However, the bioethics committee faces a number of problems, including a shortage of resources that limits the possibility of including members who have the time to work exclusively for the committee. In addition, a shortage of time available for meetings results in slow progress in the evolution of the team and insufficient follow-up of cases. The committee continues to work towards the key objectives of positioning bioethics committees in primary healthcare as a necessary part of the structure of the national health system and consistently raising awareness of the need for reflection on community bioethics and primary healthcare. The complexity of the problems and dilemmas that arise in community bioethics is amply illustrated in the following two case examples.

Case I

Unit: Family health centre
Presented by: Family healthcare team
Case: 29-year-old male patient, married, three children, frequent homosexual encounters, stated to the health team that he is HIV-positive. Asking for help, but does not wish his condition to be revealed to his wife, with whom he continues to have unprotected sexual intercourse, or to anyone else in the health centre. He is a well-known member of the community.

Background
Family: Good socio-economic conditions, owns own house and shares land with other relatives. Patient has a stable job, and spouse is a housewife. The children attend school regularly.

Family dynamics: Refers to having good family dynamics, but has had casual homosexual affairs.

Present situation: Patient has become aware that one of his casual partners is infected with HIV. Patient had blood test which is HIV-positive. Patient is asymptomatic.

Why was this case presented to the bioethics committee?

The case presents a number of key ethical questions that are distinctive in primary healthcare, in the dynamics of interpersonal relationships between service users and the health team. Is it ethically justifiable that the health team respects the confidentiality of the petitioner? Can a beneficial action generate a harmful episode? Must the health team inform the patient's spouse (a regular user of the health centre) of his HIV-positive condition, as he continues to have sexual intercourse with her without protection? Following discussion, the committee made the following recommendations:

- Provide support to the service user and avoid him disengaging from the health team, as a protective measure for him and his family.
- Always respect the confidentiality of the patient. It is the patient's, not the team's, role to inform about the HIV-positive condition of the person.
- Encourage the patient, by means of advising him, firmly and persuasively, to reveal his HIV-positive condition to his spouse and family, and follow up on this matter. Explain that this would enable his wife's HIV status to be clarified (with her informed consent) so that she might receive any necessary care.
- Teach universal precautions to the patient, specifically in relation to the sexual protection of his wife.
- Accompany and support the patient's wife and family when they so request it.
- Do not file documents openly revealing the patient's condition in the dossier; use other (medical) words such as 'immunodeficiency'.
- Provide continuous education to the team regarding HIV/AIDS, confidentiality and informed consent.

The committee's decisions and recommendations were based on the analysis of the principles of ethics. In this case all four classic principles – non-maleficence, beneficence, autonomy and justice – had been compromised. Other compromised principles were confidentiality, solidarity and protection. The principle of non-maleficence was infringed. This principle compels to not produce harm, and in this case the patient's wife was exposed to HIV infection as a consequence of the patient's performance of unprotected sexual intercourse with multiple partners without assessing the risks and consequences. Similarly, the principle of beneficence was not respected. If we consider that the family's duty is to seek the welfare of each of its members (Gracia,

1989), it is clear that in this case the patient had not acted with the welfare of his wife in mind; his actions were not in accordance with the principle of beneficence. Furthermore, the principles of autonomy and justice were implicated in this case. From a Thomistic understanding of justice, the common welfare must be considered, which is superior to individual welfare, with the result that individual actions are considered just and ultimately ethical if they are in accordance with the welfare of the community (Gracia, 1989). In this case the patient appeared to have acted in accordance with his individual welfare (exploration of his homosexual nature), and by not foreseeing the consequences of his actions he had become infected with HIV, putting his wife at a high risk of also becoming infected, and thus acting against the common welfare and infringing the principle of justice. Further support for this can be found in the contractual perspective of justice (Gracia, 1989), in which the autonomy of the individual, which in this case led him to explore his homosexual nature, has a limit that is imposed by the contract with another individual. Justice for the individual implies certain rights (to life, freedom, property, and to defend them when threatened), but the contract or pact, whose objective is social justice, identifies the common welfare. The spouse's rights were thus protected through a (matrimonial) contract in which there are two parties, but in this case the patient showed concern only for himself and acted without the free and informed consent of his wife, a condition to which he was bound by contract.

The committee concluded that it was crucial that, through advice and support, the patient be directed to communicate his HIV-positive condition to his wife. In addition, it was necessary to support the patient and his family throughout this process and during the progression of the illness. Furthermore, it was desirable, as a beneficent protective action, to respect the patient's confidentiality (as a well-known member of the community) and that of his spouse and family.

Case 2

Unit: Administration

Presented by: Director
Case: Not all professionals of the health centre agree with the Ministry of Health anti-rubella vaccination campaign. They consider that it is risky as it could produce foetal malformations in women who are not aware of their pregnancy and that it invades women's privacy, especially that of teenagers, who must be quizzed about their sexual life. A similar discussion has been held throughout the country.

Background
In an effort to avoid congenital and perinatal anomalies, the Chilean Ministry of Health has made several interventions, among them, in 1990 the introduction of the vaccine against rubella into the obligatory vaccination scheme. The purpose is to control this illness which, when it affects pregnant women, can cause severe damage to the foetus, known as Congenital Rubella Syndrome. Since the introduction of this vaccine a sustained decrease in incidence rates has been observed (MINSAL, 1999b). Nevertheless, since 1997 new outbreaks of rubella have occurred in Chile, so the Ministry of Health launched a nationwide vaccination campaign. The vaccine protects 95% of vaccinated women during their entire fertile period, and was obligatory and free. Two and a half million women aged 10–29 years were due to be vaccinated between 12 August and 10 September 1999. It is contraindicated to vaccinate feverish, immune-depressed and pregnant women, and the latter would be vaccinated after delivery (MINSAL, 1999b).

Why was this case presented to the bioethics committee?

This case presents an ethical dilemma within primary healthcare whose origin and responsibility corresponds to the public health system and its assistance network. One of the contraindications of this vaccine is pregnancy. Many teenagers carry on an active sexual life that is unknown to their families. It is likely that there are pregnant teenagers who are unaware of their condition, and others who, being aware of their pregnancy, would submit to vaccination anyway in order to keep it undisclosed. It is therefore necessary to ask about sexual activity in order to avoid risks, thus invading women's privacy, which is especially relevant to teenagers who often keep their sexual lives secret. Can an apparently beneficent action generate a harmful episode? Must professionals with a conscientious objection proceed under the Ministry of Health's orders? After discussing the case, the committee made the following recommendations:

• The health centre should proceed with the public welfare vaccination campaign as indicated by the Ministry of Health. It is desirable that this be done under the willing, well-informed consent of the recipients.
• Qualified personnel must be trained to perform the vaccinations in this campaign. Individual interviews must be carried out, without relatives or anyone else as witnesses, and with the highest respect for the privacy of the recipients, particularly that of teenagers, even when mothers and relatives insist on being informed. In any case of doubt, the person should not be vaccinated but should be sent to the midwife in order to rule out the possibility of pregnancy.

These recommendations were based on the following analysis. According to classic principles, non-maleficence could be compromised if a foetus were exposed to a contraindicated vaccine, or if a woman (teenager) suffered negative consequences as a result of her sexual secrets being disclosed. However, if administered when indicated (to non-pregnant women), the vaccination is beneficent, as it protects the developing foetus from severe damage. Autonomy also plays a part, inasmuch as private life is invaded by external paternalistic control on the part of the health authorities. The principle of justice is also implicated, since the vaccination campaign is a public health initiative that contributes to the common welfare of the population by avoiding severe congenital anomalies. The committee therefore concluded that it is desirable that public health campaigns such as this one, which involve a segment of the population highly sensitive to sexuality values, be carried out under the willing consent of recipients. Professionals who administer the vaccines must therefore be trained in advisory skills and have the utmost respect for the confidentiality of the recipient.

Conclusion

These two case studies and the examples of cases considered earlier in this chapter (see Table 6.1) provide a clear indication of the range of ethical dilemmas faced within primary healthcare on a daily basis. Crucially, it can be seen that the complexity of social interactions creates bioethical dilemmas in fields other than the clinical one. This becomes evident to primary healthcare teams when interacting with the community and its life-styles, especially when working with poor income sectors or ethnic minority groups.

Although techno-scientific conflicts are the same in Latin America as in the developed world, there are also important bioethical dilemmas arising from deficient social and cultural conditions. Life in these cases is threatened from a basic needs perspective (Velasco, 1996), more than by techno-scientific development. Therefore a strong social perspective characterises Latin American bioethics (Rosselot, 1998) and emphasises its two dimensions: one individual and private (ethics of maximum), clinically orientated, and more characteristic of developed countries (Gracia, 1989), and the other social and orientated to the common welfare, always superior to the best benefit of one individual (public ethics and ethics of minimum) (Kuttow, 2005). Or, the most complete proposal, a socialised individual bioethics, which focuses on the individual as part of a particular social context (Gracia, 1989).

We strongly believe that through dialogue and negotiation, bioethics has the potential to increase the level of understanding, tolerance and respect between people, and to strengthen the relationship between different social and cultural groups. Primary healthcare teams play an important role in this process. Therefore, we can say that there is a specific and relevant field for theoretical and practical bioethics in primary healthcare, especially in public health. Finally, we emphasise that although bioethics committees use a similar scientific method to solve ethical value conflicts, they focus on different subjects, which creates a difference between them. In the case of primary healthcare bioethics committees, the community and family bio-psychosocial approach to healthcare provides a focus. Our experience demonstrates that it is more than justified to reflect upon social and community bioethical value conflicts. Consequently, it is of great importance to develop primary care bioethics committees in each community, as a scientific means to overcome conflicts and to elaborate ethical public health protocols and policies. We would argue that it is necessary to develop public health community bioethics training programmes for primary care bioethics teams, so that they may identify vulnerable populations and community dilemmas and the ways in which they affect the work of the healthcare teams and the public health network.

Further reading

Altisent, R. (1993) 'Formación continuada en Bioética para la práctica de la medicina familiar', *JANO Medicina y Humanidades*, vol 44, no 1041, pp 57–66.

Lolas, F., Florenzano, R., Gyarmati, G. and Trejo, C. (1992) *Ciencias Sociales y Medicina. Perspectivas Latinoamericanas*, Santiago: Editorial Universitaria.

Mifsud, T. (1985) *El respeto por la vida humana (bioética). Moral de discernimiento tomo II*, Santiago: Ediciones Paulinas-CIDE.

References

Beca, J. and Kottow, M. (1996) *Orientaciones para comités de ética hospitalaria*, Documentos del programa regional de bioética OPS/OMS.

ECLAC (Economic Commission for Latin America and the Caribbean) (2007) *Statistical yearbook for Latin America and the Caribbean*, Santiago: United Nations.

Fundación Cristo Vive (2000) *Compartiendo el pan*, Santiago: Desafío Ediciones SA.

Gracia, D. (1989) *Fundamentos de Bioética*, Madrid: EUDEMA SA.

Instituto Nacional de Estadísticas (2002) *Resultados generales censo 2002*. Available at: www.ine.cl/cd2002/cuadros/1/C1_00000.pdf (accessed 8 February 2008).

Kuttow, M. (2005) *Bioética en salud pública*, Santiago: Editorial Puerto de Palo.

Ladrière, J. (2000) 'Del sentido de la bioética', *Acta Bioethica*, vol 6, no 2, pp 197–218.

Méndez, R. (2002) *El Chile que se viene*, Santiago: AFP Summa-Bansander.

MIDEPLAN (Ministerio de Planificación) (2006) *Encuesta de caracterización socioeconómica nacional CASEN 2006*. Available at: www.mideplan.cl/final/categoria.php?secid=25&catid=124 (accessed 17 February 2008).

MINSAL (Ministerio de Salud) (1999a) *Salud familiar en Chile*, Santiago: Ministerio de Salud.

MINSAL (1999b) *Fundamentos técnicos de la campaña de vacunación antirubéola*. Available at: http://epi.minsal.cl/epi/html/public/rubeola/anttec.pdf (accessed 2 February 2008).

MINSAL (2006) *Objetivos sanitarios para la década 2000–2010. Evaluación a mitad de período*, Santiago: Ministerio de Salud.

Rosselot, E. (1998) 'Proyecciones bioéticas de algunos aspectos de la realidad económico-social y medico-social', *Cuadernos Médico Sociales*, vol 39, no 1, pp 80–6.

Solari, M. (2003) *Ámbito de la bioética en la atención primaria de salud*, Tesis de Magíster, Facultad de Medicina, Universidad de Chile.

Thompson, M. (2000) *Ethics*, London: Hodder Headline.

United Nations (1992) Conferencia de las Naciones Unidas sobre el Medio Ambiente y el Desarrollo, *Río de Janeiro, República Federativa del Brasil â junio de 1992*. Available at: www2.medioambiente.gov.ar/acuerdos/convênciones/rio92/Default.htm (accessed 10 February 2008).

Velasco, D. (1996) *La dimensión social de la bioética, elementos para un diálogo*, Santiago: ILADES.

WHO (World Health Organization) (1978) *Declaration of Alma-Ata, International Conference on Primary Health Care, Alma-Ata, USSR, 6–12 September 1978*. Available at: www.inclusion-ia.org/espa%F1ol/Norm/almaata_declaration.pdf (accessed 10 February 2008).

Zurro, M. and Pérez, C. (2000) *Compendio de Atención Primaria*, España: Ediciones Harcourt SA.

SEVEN

Unlinked anonymous blood testing for public health purposes: an ethical dilemma?

Jessica Datta and Anthony Kessell

A s has already been discussed, public health ethics centres on a problematic triad consisting of governments, the population and individuals. This triad is the focus of this chapter, with particular reference to the testing of blood for HIV for research purposes. This raises a number of important issues concerning such things as informed consent, the use of human tissue and how the information gained might legitimately be used.

Introduction

In this chapter we describe unlinked anonymous blood testing for human immunodeficiency virus (HIV) and other diseases, and examine the ethical issues associated with this system of seroprevalence testing. We argue that the views of participants have been missing from ethical debates about seroprevalence monitoring, and propose that the issue of informed consent for inclusion in such programmes should be revisited. We introduce our own current scientific research which explores this issue.

A discussion about the ethics of unlinked anonymous testing of blood should be placed within wider contemporary debates in the arenas of public health, clinical medicine and medical research. The first such debate focuses on the balance between individuals' rights and the appropriate role of government in infringing on those rights for broader public health interests or concerns. Connected to this is the extent to which the traditional doctor–patient relationship extends to public health, and the degree of public health paternalism that is acceptable. The second debate centres on the boundaries of informed consent in medical research, particularly in relation to the use of human tissue, and the extent to which information contained in medical records can be utilised for research purposes.

In relation to the first debate, there has been strong criticism of government in recent times, particularly in the mass media, for its 'nanny state' approach to interventions in, for example, the areas of smoking, alcohol and diet. More recently the notion of 'stewardship' (Jochelson, 2005) in public health rejects these negative associations, and advocates that government should have a role to play in protecting the health of citizens, preventing them from harming themselves or others, and promoting healthy behaviour. In this view, public health interventions should not be thought of as unwanted restrictions imposed by a 'nanny' on powerless children, but as actions that favour both individuals and society more widely, as prescribed by a 'steward' administering and protecting citizens' interests.[1] Although this approach may impose some limitations on individuals' liberty, these are balanced by the associated benefits. The Nuffield Council on Bioethics, for example, in advocating a 'stewardship model' for public health, argues that the state should act as steward both to individuals and to the population as a whole, but that individuals' personal choices should also be taken into account. This model "gives expression to the obligation on states to seek to provide conditions that allow people to be healthy, especially in relation to reducing health inequalities" (Nuffield Council on Bioethics, 2007).

A parallel and connected discussion has been going on in the field of clinical medicine over a similar period, and has questioned the paternalism of the medical profession towards patients, who have traditionally been seen as passive recipients of treatment. This model has gradually been replaced with a more equal relationship, in which patients are seen as active citizens, participating in healthcare as both discerning service users and experts in their own right. Meanwhile, medical research has increasingly been regulated by research ethics committees that aim to protect potential research participants from unnecessary harm (Garrard and Dawson, 2005).

Unlinked anonymous blood testing is carried out in order to provide information about the prevalence and spread of particular infectious diseases in a population. According to the Department of Health, "the data obtained are used to target and evaluate health promotion, to inform estimates of the numbers requiring treatment and care in the future, and to plan services for those affected by HIV and AIDS" (Department of Health, 2008). Testing is therefore not in itself a public health 'intervention', but a prerequisite for such an intervention. This chapter explores whether ethical issues pertaining to the programme should be reviewed in light of these evolving debates.

The unlinked anonymous serosurveillance programme in England and Wales

The Unlinked Anonymous Prevalence Monitoring Programme (UAPMP) was set up in 1989 by the Department of Health, began its screening work in January 1990 and is ongoing. The programme was developed in response to concerns about the spread of HIV during the 1980s and, in particular, the demand for high-quality evidence on its prevalence. Despite initial opposition from both members of the medical establishment and politicians to unlinked, anonymous serosurveillance, the methodology gained political acceptability in 1989 when Kenneth Clarke, then Secretary of State for Health, gave it his support (Berridge, 1996). The programme was funded as a pilot project for two years by the Medical Research Council, and has since been funded by the Department of Health.

The primary aim of the programme has been described as "to measure trends in HIV infection among those whose behaviour and social networks are associated with increased risk" (Department of Health, 1998). However, another important objective is to assess prevalence in the wider population. The specific objectives of the programme are shown in Box 7.1.

The programme is managed by the Health Protection Agency (HPA)[2] (formerly the Public Health Laboratory Service) and the Institute of Child Health, University of London. In order to meet its aims, the programme uses data collected from three ongoing surveys to measure the proportion of individuals within the general population, and within subgroups of the population, infected with HIV at any given point or period in time. The programme findings are for England and Wales. Health Protection Scotland (HPS) coordinates data collection in Scotland.

The principles of the programme

The principles underpinning seroprevalence surveillance are very different from those of case finding. Case finding involves testing to identify individuals who are positive for HIV antibodies (HIV+). In contrast, seroprevalence surveys do *not* aim to identify individuals who are HIV+, but instead use blood specimens which are unnamed (anonymous) and which cannot be traced back to the individual (unlinked), through the irreversible removal of personal identifiers and batch processing in laboratories. This means, of course, that individuals whose blood is tested positive for HIV cannot be contacted or informed.

Box 7.1: Objectives of the Unlinked Anonymous Prevalence Monitoring Programme

- To monitor the prevalence of, and associated risks for, HIV infection in accessible groups of those adults whose risk behaviour makes them vulnerable to infection, such as attenders at genito-urinary medicine clinics and injecting drug users.
- To measure, through serosurveillance of accessible groups, the impact of HIV infection on those who are less vulnerable behaviourally and are more broadly representative of the adult population.
- To monitor closely the prevalence of HIV infection in London and to recognise emerging problems elsewhere.
- To measure the effectiveness of voluntary confidential testing strategies for clinical diagnosis of HIV infections.
- In combination with other data, to provide estimates of the total numbers of HIV-infected persons and assist in projecting future numbers of persons with severe HIV disease who will require care.
- To use specimens gathered by the programme to measure the prevalence of, and associated risk factors for, other infections of public health or scientific importance.
- To make available scientific programme data in a timely and accessible form so as to inform the targeting of health promotion, the assessment of the effectiveness of preventive measures, and the planning of medical and social services for those affected by HIV.

Source: Department of Health (1998).

The UAPMP uses data from seroprevalence surveys, as well as reports from clinics on numbers of individuals who are HIV+ (which derive from case finding), to build up a picture of prevalence in the population at a particular time. The principles of the unlinked anonymous method of seroprevalence are presented in Box 7.2.

Box 7.2: Principles of the Unlinked Anonymous Prevalence Monitoring Programme

- Necessary clinical specimens of usual amount
- Original clinical test not compromised
- Unlinked and made anonymous before HIV test
- Restricted data set to prevent indirect identification
- Access to named HIV testing for target population
- Valid study design.

Source: Gill et al (1989).

Explicit consent from those whose blood is used in the programme is not required (apart from injecting drug users who provide saliva samples voluntarily) and clinicians do not necessarily inform patients about their inclusion. Information about the programme in the form of leaflets and/or a poster should be displayed in clinics participating in the programme, and patients should therefore be able to choose whether to opt out if they prefer. In practice, however, many patients may not know about the programme and, as it may not be explicitly mentioned by clinicians, are not able to express their choice to opt out.

The blood tested in the unlinked anonymous surveys is blood left over from routine tests. Although these residual specimens are unnamed and unlinked (from the individual), certain demographic information is retained. In the Unlinked Anonymous Dried Blood Spots survey, for example, the year of a baby's birth and residence information are initially retained. In selected regions, linkage is made with birth registration data – hospital of birth, age of mother and parents' country of birth. However, this linkage is temporary and the blood spots are permanently unlinked from all identifiers and anonymised before testing takes place (The UK Collaborative Group for HIV and STI Surveillance, 2007).

The programme's surveys

Three unlinked anonymous surveys are used to monitor the prevalence and spread of HIV; two of these include service users at higher risk of HIV infection, and the third those who are less vulnerable. The three surveys are the Unlinked Anonymous Genito-urinary Medicine clinic survey, which uses residual blood taken for syphilis serology; the Unlinked Anonymous Dried Blood Spots survey, which tests residual neonatal blood spots taken for routine screening for material anti-HIV antibodies; and the Unlinked Anonymous Injecting Drug Users (IDUs) survey, which uses voluntary samples collected from IDUs who attend specialist agencies. A number of other surveys provide additional information.

The HPA's recent annual report on HIV and other sexually transmitted infections lists the data sources used (The UK Collaborative Group for HIV and STI Surveillance, 2007). These include the Annual Survey of Prevalent HIV Infections Diagnosed (SOPHID) on numbers of people using HIV-related care, and the National Study of HIV in Pregnancy and Childhood (NSHPC), which includes confidential reports of HIV-infected pregnant women, infants born to infected women and HIV-infected children. The largest number of samples derives from the infant dried blood spots. To date, the unlinked anonymous surveys have tested around ten million blood samples.

The value of the programme

The findings of the unlinked anonymous programme appear to be valued by researchers, public health professionals, policy makers and health practitioners. They provide "minimally biased estimates" (Nicoll et al, 2000) on the prevalence of HIV which are more accurate and of higher quality than those provided by an aggregate of cases identified in the population. It has been described as "an essential component" (Nicoll et al, 2000) in the range of surveillance methodologies used for the monitoring of sexually acquired infections.

In particular, the programme has been able to track changes in the size and characteristics of the HIV+ population and to identify a sizeable minority of people in this population who remain undiagnosed and who, therefore, are not receiving treatment. In 2006, data from the unlinked anonymous programme provided evidence that approximately 21,600 people (31% of the total of the estimated 73,000 people living with HIV in the United Kingdom) remained undiagnosed (The UK Collaborative Group for HIV and STI Surveillance, 2007). Findings from the surveys, in conjunction with data on the number of positive named tests for HIV, have influenced testing policy at genito-urinary medicine (GUM) clinics. The National Strategy for Sexual Health and HIV target of offering an HIV test to all new GUM clinic users, for example, was informed by concern about the large numbers of undiagnosed individuals attending clinics (Department of Health, 2002).

A component of an evaluation of the unlinked anonymous programme (Kessel and Watts, 1999; 2001) aimed to measure the degree to which it met its seventh objective, namely to provide data to target health promotion, to assess the effectiveness of preventative measures, and to plan services. A large majority (87.3%) of respondents to the survey of health authority staff (Kessel and Watts, 2001) reported finding the information provided by the programme "useful in general" while over two-thirds (67.3%) reported finding it "useful for targeting health promotion". One commentator has argued that the availability of the information derived from the programme allows service providers "to shape and refine clinical practice to the benefit of others", and to "focus resources" effectively (Pinching, 2000). However, there is little published evidence evaluating the programme's practical usefulness (or otherwise) to public health professionals, service commissioners or providers, or comparing the effectiveness of the programme for planning services with that of other countries which do not use unlinked anonymous surveillance systems.

Ethical issues

There are two main ethical issues associated with the programme and which have concerned commentators. The first is the question of informed consent by participants for inclusion in the programme (Trouet, 2004). The second is that, because the residual blood tested is unlinked from the individual who gave the sample, it is not possible to inform someone if their blood tests positive for HIV (de Zulueta, 2000). The following section introduces the ethical approach of principlism in relation to unlinked anonymous seroprevalence. We then discuss informed consent both in a historical context and in the light of more recent developments in relationships between patients (and the general public) and the health service. Evidence about patients' understanding of the unlinking process is also considered.

Principlism and unlinked anonymous seroprevalence programmes

Most of the ethical debate about unlinked anonymous testing for HIV has taken place, explicitly or implicitly, within a framework of the four principles of bioethics (principlism) advocated primarily by the American philosophers Beauchamp and Childress (Beauchamp and Childress, 1994), but now an established part of mainstream medical ethics (Engelhardt, 1994). The four principles are respect for individual autonomy, beneficence, non-maleficence and justice.

Principlism asserts that any medico-ethical dilemma can be analysed by exploring and balancing these principles. For seroprevalence monitoring of HIV, the argument runs that the benefits to society from unlinked anonymous testing for HIV outweigh any compromise of the other principles and therefore the policy should be adopted (Bayer, 1993; Dunn et al, 1995). It is helpful to look briefly at each principle to appreciate this balancing act.

The principle of respect for autonomy asserts the importance of individual self-determination over one's body or body parts. Informed consent should therefore be given before testing a blood sample for HIV and, as this is usually not explicitly the case with unlinked anonymous testing, the principle is compromised. The dilemma for policy makers and scientists is that the epidemiological quality and usefulness of the data collected by the programme might be compromised if each participant were asked to provide individual consent (not to mention the extra time this would add to consultations).

The principle of non-maleficence stresses the duty not to harm others. In past debates, weight of opinion has been that unlinked anonymous testing for HIV does the tested individual no harm, as their situation is unchanged by the testing, and voluntary testing remains an available option (Buehler et al, 1994). However, individuals may feel harmed in a broader sense if they discover they have not been informed and that therefore their views have not been respected (Kopelman, 1994).

It is the principle of beneficence that most strongly supports unlinked anonymous testing for HIV. As the philosopher John Stuart Mill stated 150 years ago, "the only purpose for which power can be rightfully exercised over any member of a civilised community, against his will, is to prevent harm to others" (Mill, 1975). It could be argued that "harm to others" can be prevented by high-quality information about the spread of a serious disease and that therefore this principle supports the unlinked anonymous programme. The principles of non-maleficence and beneficence represent a spectrum between coercion (for example, quarantining those infected by a particular disease) and a liberal approach to public health (for example, providing information on the dangers of smoking). Unlinked anonymous blood testing, which provides public health information and is relatively non-invasive for participating individuals, could be said to be at the beneficence end of this spectrum.

Informed consent and ethics: a changing debate

Respect for autonomy is the principle that is most likely to be jeopardised by a programme of unlinked anonymous blood testing, since informed consent is not deemed necessary for an individual's blood to be included in the programme. In debates held in the late 1980s and early 1990s – chronicled by Berridge (1996) – the opposing views of those who were concerned about patient consent and those who felt that the priority was to control what was seen as an epidemic were publicly aired. These views are illustrated by the very different positions taken by two leading figures.

Professor Ian Kennedy, an academic ethicist at the time, argued that "under *no* circumstances can blood samples be tested without informed consent" (Bayer et al, 1990). On the other hand, Professor Richard Doll, chair of the Medical Research Council/Department of Health and Social Services (MRC/DHSS) subcommittee on the epidemiology of AIDS, and James Gowan, secretary of the MRC, asked "how it can be unethical is incomprehensible, as it can do no possible harm to anyone and could do much good" (Doll, 1987). The programme did eventually go ahead and, since its inception, there has been limited debate about the ethics of the programme in England and Wales. However, it is important to note that some countries have explicitly rejected unlinked anonymous testing on ethical grounds.

Since the programme's establishment, informed consent has emerged as "the ethical touchstone of medical research, and is now enshrined in practice and a range of international guidelines as one of the main preconditions of medical research" (Cassell and Young, 2002). The expectation that patients should be provided with clear, accessible information and should sign a detailed consent form before taking part in research has become a norm for both medical and social research. Yet, informed consent has not been deemed necessary for the inclusion of an individual's blood sample in the unlinked anonymous programme. There are several reasons for this. First, it has been argued that results may be biased if each individual whose blood is used is asked for explicit consent as it is possible, for example, that those more at risk of infection might be more likely than others to decline to take part, and this would adversely affect the epidemiological usefulness of the data. Second, the need for clinicians to explain the programme to individual patients and to elicit signed consent would be time consuming and therefore expensive. Third, the inclusion of a sample of unlinked and anonymised 'leftover' blood in the programme "ranks low on the intervention ladder" (Nuffield Council on Bioethics, 2007), and is therefore not seen as significant enough to demand informed consent.

Much has changed, however, since the unlinked anonymous programme was developed in the late 1980s. At that time the feared AIDS epidemic was seen as a public health emergency, there was no treatment available, transmission from mother to unborn child was not preventable, and the stigma and discrimination associated with the infection were more overt than is currently the case in the UK. As previously discussed, in the same period there has been a shift in relationships between the medical profession, scientists, patients of the health service and the public more widely. However, this changing context has not brought about any substantial alteration to the unlinked anonymous programme regarding the issue of consent. Prominent bioethicists have argued that "it is acceptable to collect and use anonymised data for assessing and predicting trends in infectious disease without consent, as long as any invasion of privacy is reduced as far as possible" (Nuffield Council on Bioethics, 2007), and new legislation does not contest this view. Although the 2004 Human Tissue

Act makes "consent the fundamental principle underpinning the lawful retention and use of bodyparts, organs and tissues from the living", it exempts "surplus or 'residual' tissue" taken from living patients which is leftover from diagnostic or surgical procedures" for use in public health monitoring (Department of Health, 2004).

Patients' knowledge and understanding of blood testing

Rather than being asked for consent for the use of their 'leftover' blood, the population groups whose samples are routinely included in the programme (primarily the mothers of newborn babies and users of GUM services) are supposed to receive prior notification of the programme. This means that they should have access to printed literature (a poster and/or leaflets produced in a number of languages) in the clinic or ward that informs them of the programme and lets them know that they can opt out if they wish. The poster, produced by the Department of Health in 2000, explains that inclusion of a person's blood in the programme "does not mean you personally are having an HIV test", because identifying information is removed from the sample before it is tested. The accompanying leaflet offers advice on where to go for an HIV test and provides contact details for the National AIDS Helpline, thus offering patients the opportunity to take a named test to find out their HIV status (Department of Health, 2000).

One concern about the system of 'prior notification' is that patients may not see posters or leaflets in the clinic, or may not understand the significance of the information included. Opinions expressed by respondents in our current research suggest that information is not always displayed prominently and, in some cases, is not available at all. The plethora of posters adorning clinic walls may dissuade patients from reading them and could mean that they are unable to easily differentiate which posters are relevant to them.

Lack of public awareness about the programme is evidenced by findings from a survey carried out in 1998 (Kessel et al, 2000) which suggest that a minority of those in the general population know about the programme. Fewer than a third (31.5%) of a randomly selected sample of 1,845 people aged over 16 reported being aware of its existence. Those aged 25–44 years were more likely to be aware than those in younger or older age groups. Preliminary findings from a new study carried out by the authors of this chapter suggest that a large majority of users of two sexual health clinics – both of which contribute blood samples to the Unlinked Anonymous Genito-urinary Medicine clinic survey – are unaware of the programme.

What happens to the blood?

There has been relatively little literature published on patients' understanding of the processes in blood testing, or how taken or 'leftover' blood is used. Pfeffer and Laws (Pfeffer and Laws, 2006) conducted 19 focus groups in a London teaching hospital with patients using obstetric and gynaecology services, hospital staff (healthcare professionals and pathologists) and the general public, focusing on their knowledge of venepuncture and the uses of blood taken for testing. They found that there was considerable uncertainty about what happens to blood following its production. They report that, although participants thought research using blood taken explicitly for that purpose was of potential benefit, research using 'leftover' blood was seen as illegitimate, "conjur[ing] up fantasies drawn from horror movies and books about evil doctors and scientists" (Pfeffer and Laws, 2006).

The same study found that in a reported discussion about the use of 'leftover' samples a majority of participants argued that they would want to know what research was being carried out and be given the opportunity to consent. However, a minority said they would not mind what happened to such samples and expressed great confidence in the health service to "do the right thing" (Pfeffer and Laws, 2006). In conclusion, the authors describe 'leftover' blood as an anomaly – participants thought of it as "an excess (waste), a challenge (to use wisely), or a crime (illegitimate research)" (Pfeffer and Laws, 2006). These findings suggest that patients and members of the general public are ill-informed about the uses made of blood and that, in ignorance, they attribute a number of different scenarios to what actually happens to it.

Conclusions: an ongoing ethical dilemma?

There is clearly an ethical dilemma regarding the issue of consent and unlinked anonymous blood testing. However, it is worth considering how significant the dilemma really is. Although it can be argued that the use of 'leftover' blood from diagnostic tests for surveillance or research purposes is not high on the intervention ladder and that its inclusion does not directly harm those whose blood is tested, respect for individual autonomy suggests that consent should be sought from those whose blood is included in the programme.

Some commentators argue that even anonymised tissue should not be used without consent. Trouet (2004), for example, believes that the use of such material is in contravention of Article 22 of the Convention on Human Rights and Biomedicine (Council of Europe, 1997). The article states that "when in the course of an intervention any part of a human body is removed, it may be stored and used for a purpose other than that for which it was removed, only if this is done in conformity with appropriate information and consent procedures" (Trouet, 2004). Trouet suggests that patients' assessment of the personal value attributed to tissue may differ from that of researchers.

In recent years commentators have argued that patients of a publicly supported healthcare system like the National Health Service have a moral duty to participate in scientific research (Harris, 2005; Evans, 2007), although most do not go so far as to articulate that such participation should be mandatory in practice (Shapshay and Pimple, 2007). Our current survey of over 400 users of two GUM clinics has provisionally found that a large majority of respondents (89%) agree that people should have a responsibility to take part in research studies, and the same proportion would agree to the use of their blood in unlinked anonymous seroprevalence testing. However, when asked about the question of consent, 74% believed that they should be asked to consent before their blood is used for public health surveillance. The way forward perhaps is to ensure that patients – and the public more widely – are informed of the existence, purposes and value of disease surveillance arrangements (Cassell and Young, 2002) and to investigate alternative arrangements for gaining consent which are not unnecessarily cumbersome or likely to create bias among those who agree that their blood be used.

The issue of consent in seroprevalence surveillance remains an important instrument to gauge and probe the moral direction of public health policies more broadly. Debate continues around whether public health programmes are morally valid in embracing the more paternalistic 'nanny' role, or should instead take on a more Kantian stewardship function. Examining why different countries have adopted different moral positions in relation to seroprevalence surveillance will help to illuminate our understanding of how moral direction becomes embedded in public health policies and practice.

Notes

[1] It is interesting that in this discourse 'nanny' (female) is seen as negative and 'steward' (male) as positive, when both are servants employed to manage and protect.

[2] It was previously managed by the Communicable Disease Surveillance Centre, part of the Public Health Laboratory Service, which ceased to exist in 2003.

References

Bayer, R. (1993) 'The ethics of blinded HIV surveillance testing', *American Journal of Public Health*, vol 83, pp 496–7.

Bayer, R., Lumey, L.H. and Wan, L. (1990) 'The American, British and Dutch responses to unlinked anonymous HIV seroprevalence studies: an international comparison', *AIDS*, vol 4, pp 283–90.

Beauchamp, T.L. and Childress, J.F. (1994) *Principles of biomedical ethics*, New York: Oxford University Press.

Berridge, V. (1996) *AIDS in the UK: The making of policy 1981–1994*, Oxford: Oxford University Press.

Buehler, J.W., Petersen, L.R., Ward, J.W. and Valdiserri, R.O. (1994) 'Defending HIV seroprevalence surveys', *American Journal of Public Health*, vol. 84, pp 319–20.

Cassell, J. and Young, A. (2002) 'Why we should not seek individual informed consent for participation in health services research', *Journal of Medical Ethics*, vol 28, pp 313–17.

Council of Europe (1997) *Convention for the protection of human rights and dignity of the human being with regard to the application of biology and medicine: convention on human rights and biomedicine*, European Treaty Series, no 164.

De Zulueta, P. (2000) 'The ethics of anonymised HIV testing of pregnant women: a reappraisal', *Journal of Medical Ethics*, vol 26, pp 16–21.

Department of Health (1998) *Prevalence of HIV in England and Wales in 1997: Annual report of the Unlinked Anonymous Prevalence Monitoring Programme*, London: Department of Health

Department of Health (2000) *If you are having a blood sample taken ...*, Patient information leaflet, London: Department of Health.

Department of Health (2002) *The national strategy for sexual health and HIV: Implementation action plan*, London: Department of Health.

Department of Health (2004) *The Human Tissue Act 2004: New legislation on human organs and tissue*, London: Department of Health.

Department of Health (2008) *Unlinked Anonymous Prevalence Monitoring Programme*, London: Department of Health.

Doll, R. (1987) 'A proposal for doing prevalence studies of AIDS', *British Medical Journal*, vol 294, pp 443–4.

Dunn, D.T., Nicoll, A., Holland, F.J. and Davison, C.F. (1995) 'How much paediatric HIV infection could be prevented by antenatal HIV testing', *Journal of Medical Screening*, vol 2, pp 35–40.

Engelhardt, H.T.J. (1994) *The foundations of bioethics*, Oxford: Oxford University Press.

Evans, H.M. (2007) 'Do patients have duties?', *Journal of Medical Ethics*, vol 33, pp 689–94.

Garrard, E. and Dawson, A. (2005) 'What is the role of the Research Ethics Committee? Paternalism, inducements, and harm in research ethics', *Journal of Medical Ethics*, vol 31, pp 419–23.

Gill, O.N., Adler, M.W. and Day, N.E. (1989) 'Monitoring the prevalence of HIV: foundations for a programme of unlinked anonymous testing in England and Wales', *British Medical Journal*, vol 299, pp 1295–7.

Harris, J. (2005) 'Scientific research is a moral duty', *Journal of Medical Ethics*, vol 31, pp 242–8.

Jochelson, K. (2005) 'Nanny or steward? The role of government in public health', King's Fund Working Paper, London: King's Fund.

Kessel, A.S. and Watts, C.J. (1999) 'Usefulness of information from the Unlinked Anonymous Prevalence Monitoring Programme for HIV in England and Wales: survey of planners of HIV/AIDS services', *International Journal of STD and AIDS*, vol 10, pp 808–11.

Kessel, A.S. and Watts, C.J. (2001) 'Evaluation of the unlinked anonymous prevalence monitoring programme for HIV in England and Wales: science, ethics and health policy', *Medical Science Monitor*, vol 7, pp 1052–63.

Kessel, A., Watts, C. and Weiss, H.A. (2000) 'Bad blood? Survey of public's views on unlinked anonymous testing of blood for HIV and other diseases', *British Medical Journal*,, vol 320, pp 90–1.

Kopelman, L.M. (1994) 'Informed consent and anonymous tissue samples: the case of HIV seroprevalence studies', *Journal of Medicine and Philosophy*, vol 19, pp 525–52.

Mill, J.S. (1975) 'On liberty', in J.S. Mill, *Three essays: On liberty, representative government, the subjection of women*, Oxford: Oxford University Press, pp 5–141.

Nicoll, A., Gill, O.N., Peckham, C., Ades, A.E., Parry, J., Mortimer, P., Goldberg, D., Noone, A., Bennett, D. and Catchpole, M. (2000) 'The public health applications of unlinked anonymous seroprevalence monitoring for HIV in the United Kingdom', *International Journal of Epidemiology*, vol 29, 1–10.

Nuffield Council on Bioethics (2007) *Public health: ethical issues*, London: Nuffield Council on Bioethics.

Pfeffer, N. and Laws, S. (2006) '"It's only a blood test": what people know and think about venepuncture and blood', *Social Science & Medicine*, vol 62, pp 3011–23.

Pinching, A.J. (2000) 'The ethics of anonymised HIV testing of pregnant women: a reappraisal – commentary', *Journal of Medical Ethics*, vol 26, pp 22–24.

Shapshay, S. and Pimple, K.D. (2007) 'Participation in biomedical research is an imperfect moral duty: a response to John Harris', *Journal of Medical Ethics*, vol 33, pp 414–17.

The UK Collaborative Group for HIV and STI Surveillance (2007) 'Testing times. HIV and other sexually transmitted infections in the United Kingdom', London: Health Protection Agency, Centre for Infections.

Trouet, C. (2004) 'New European guidelines for the use of stored human biological materials in biomedical research', *Journal of Medical Ethics*, vol 30, pp 99–103.

EIGHT

Constructing the obesity epidemic: loose science, money and public health

Alison Hann and Stephen Peckham

As Cribb has commented (Chapter Two, this volume), the way in which public health problems are constructed can have value judgements embedded in them, and this can feed into policies and practices. This chapter looks at the way obesity has been constructed as a public health 'problem'. It is argued that not only does it contain masked value judgements, but also the evidence base is weak. The result is a policy which is potentially 'harmful' to those individuals labelled as obese.

Introduction

According to the World Health Organization, we are in the grip of "globesity" that is "taking over" the world (WHO, 2008). The language used here is both interesting and typical of the language used in many official (and unofficial) documents discussing obesity. Obesity is often presented as a crisis for the economy and well-being of states, as well as a very serious health risk to the individual.[1] It would be difficult to miss the note of panic that invariably creeps in. WHO claims that obesity will overwhelm both developed and underdeveloped countries and that unless immediate action is taken "millions will suffer". Participants at the world obesity conference in New Orleans in 2007 warned that "the global epidemic of obesity is completely out of control", adding that "health care services ... will not be able to cope" (Lichtarowicz, 2007). Reporting on the conference, CBS News called obesity an "international scourge", a "pandemic that threatens to overwhelm every countries [*sic*] health system", while Professor Paul Zimmet told delegates at the opening of the 2006 international congress on obesity in Australia that obesity was "an insidious creeping pandemic" which was "engulfing the entire world". The UK Department of Health takes the matter seriously enough to refer to obesity as an "epidemic" and "the most significant public and personal health challenge facing our society" (DH, 2008). The recently announced UK strategy on obesity will cost £372 million, with a further £75 million aimed at childhood obesity (DH, 2008), and the Secretary of State for Health sees the issue as very straightforward: "the problem is simple – we eat too much and we do too little exercise". The government's Chief Scientific Adviser and the head of the Government Office for Science's think tank Foresight has estimated that obesity will "cost some £45.5 billion a year by 2050" (Government Office for Science, 2007).

However the story of the obesity problem is framed, it is clear that in many of the articles, scientific journals, newspaper stories and official documents, obesity represents a looming global health disaster which will eventually affect everyone in one way or another. In addition, it is a story that contains many elements of moral judgement. As seen above, people simply eat too much and exercise too little – they are either gluttonous or slothful (or both). Advice on how people should address their weight problem is framed by concepts of 'normality'. This is demonstrated in guidance for the public issued by the National Institute for Health and Clinical Excellence (NICE, 2008) (Figure 8.1).

This chapter takes issue with some of these truths, and furthermore looks at the moral questions surrounding a public health policy that rests on equivocal evidence, sustains the stigma against overweight and obese persons, and has a part to play in the causation of untold human misery. The chapter highlights how these issues and resultant uncertainties also create ethical dilemmas for public health practice.

What is 'known' about obesity

The WHO claims that obesity is the fastest growing disease in the world and, according to its guidelines for measuring obesity (BMI equal to or greater than 30), the UK has the highest prevalence of obesity (23% of the population) in Europe (WHO, 2007). Within the UK, the obesity prevalence rates are 24% in Scotland and Northern Ireland, 23% in England and somewhat lower at 18% in Wales. The prevalence is slightly higher in socially disadvantaged groups and in women as compared with men (23.1% and 24.8% respectively) (NHS, 2006). There are distinct differences in prevalence between ethnic groups. The Health Survey for England 2004 found that people from most minority ethnic groups had lower obesity rates (Bangladeshi men 6%, Chinese men 6%, Chinese women 8%), although black Caribbean women (32%), African (39%) and Pakistani women (28%) and Irish (25%) and Black Caribbean men (25%) had the highest obesity prevalence rates (NHS, 2006).

Figure 8.1: NICE Clinical Guideline on Obesity

Recommendations for the public

Staying a healthy weight improves health and reduces the risk of diseases associated with being overweight or obese, such as coronary heart diseases, Type 2 diabetes, osteoarthritis and some cancers. Health professionals should reinforce the messages in this section.

General advice
- Check your weight or waist measurement every now and then, or keep track of the 'fit' of your clothes, to make sure you are not gaining weight.
- Discuss any concerns about your (or your family's) diet, activity levels or weight with a GP or practice nurse, health visitor, school nurse or pharmacist.
- *Adults:* use a weight loss programme (such as a commercial or self-help group, book or website) only if it is based on a balanced diet, encourages regular exercise, and expects weight loss of no more than 0.5–1kg per week. People with certain medical conditions – such as Type 2 diabetes, heart failure or uncontrolled hypertension or angina – should check with their GP's surgery or hospital specialist before starting a weight loss programme.

How to have a healthy balanced diet
- Base meals on starchy foods such as potatoes, bread, rice and pasta, choosing wholegrain where possible.
- Eat plenty of fibre-rich-foods – such as oats, beans, peas, lentils, grains, seeds, fruit and vegetables, as well as wholegrain bread, brown rice and pasta.
- Eat at least five portions of fruit and vegetables a day in place of foods higher in fat and calories.
- Eat a low-fat diet, and avoid increasing your fat and/or calorie intake.
- Eat as little as possible of: fried foods; drinks and confectionary high in added sugars; and other food and drinks high in fat and sugar, such as some take-away and fast foods.
- Eat breakfast.
- Watch the portion size of meals and snacks, and how often you are eating.
- Avoid taking in too many calories in the form of alcohol.
- *Children and young people:* should have regular meals in a pleasant and sociable environment with no distractions (such as television); parents and carers should join them as often as possible.

How to keep physically active
- Make activities you enjoy – such as walking, cycling, swimming, aerobics or gardening – part of your everyday life. Small everyday changes can make a difference.
- At work, take the stairs instead of the lift, or go for a walk at lunchtime.
- Avoid sitting too long in front of the television, computer or playing video games.
- *For children:*
- gradually reduce the time they are sitting in front of a screen
- encourage games that involve running around, such as skipping, dancing or ball games
- be more active as a family, by walking or cycling to school, going to the park, or swimming
- encourage children to take part in sport inside and outside school.

Source: NICE (2008, p 11)

According to NHS statistics (NHS, 2006), obese women are almost 13 times more likely to develop Type 2 diabetes than non–obese women, while obese men are nearly five times more likely to develop the illness. There were 2,749 Finished Consultant Episodes (FCEs) with a primary diagnosis of obesity in England in 2005/06, compared with 787 FCEs in 1996/97 (NHS, 2006). Where there was a secondary diagnosis of obesity, there were 62,708 FCEs in 2005/06, as compared with 21,257 in 1996/97. Almost 871,000 prescription items were dispensed in 2005 for the treatment of obesity, as compared with just over 127,000 prescription items in 1999 (an increase of 585%) (NHS, 2006). Surgery for obesity has been steadily rising since the mid 1990s, with the number of bariatric surgical procedures increasing from under 100 in 1997 to nearly 350 in 2004 and 6,000 in 2007. Moreover, surgeons suggest that 10 times the number of operations should be undertaken in the UK, including extending the current limit on access to such operations from people with a BMI of 35 to people with a BMI of over 25 (Ells et al, 2007; Randerson, 2008).

The Wanless Report (2004) estimated that the cost of treating obesity in the UK was £9.4 million in 1998 and the additional cost of treating attributable diseases a further £470 million. Wanless estimated that the cost to the economy as a whole by 2010 would be £3.6 billion, while the House of Commons Health Select Committee estimated that the cost to the NHS in 2002 was £1 billion (Health Select Committee, 2004).

These figures show the increasing burden on the NHS and the economy from the obesity epidemic. These figures are well known and are commonly attributed to a number of causative factors. First, people eat too much, and too much of the wrong things. Second, people have become far too sedentary and do not play enough sport or do enough walking. Furthermore, the situation is getting worse. This is often based on the idea that this is contrary to the past.

We just do not exercise enough ...

In the case of lack of exercise, a number of strands need to be examined more closely and critically. First, the idea that modern life (particularly urban life) produces weak minds and lazy bodies is not new. Indeed it has been a cornerstone of what Goldstein (1992) calls "the health movement" for at least 150 years, but as Gard and Wright (2005) point out, it is important to bear in mind that "Western populations have never been what they used to be"(p 28). For example, the 1950s is often seen as a time before society "let itself go", as Boreham and Riddoch (2003) comment:

> Today's 50–60-year-old adult is likely to have walked or cycled to school, played for hours outside the house, was not distracted by too much television, and eventually, walked to work – which was probably a manual job. So any baseline physical activity or fitness may be misleading as we know that there has been an inexorable decrease in activity levels in all sectors of our society over the last 50 years. (p 22)

This "inexorable decrease" in activity is difficult to support with empirical evidence, especially when differences between social classes are taken into account. Activity levels for individuals are notoriously difficult to measure, particularly if compared with periods of time in the past. For example, when asked about physical activity, people may remember that they attended a keep-fit class, but not how many flights of stairs they climb at work, how far they walk when shopping or how long they spend gardening. Even in rigorous studies, there is no agreement over the amount (or intensity) of exercise needed to provide individual health benefits and weight loss. The situation is complicated further by controversy over whether it is physical activity itself or the weight loss caused by physical activity that confers health benefits. It is worth noting that there was a time when virtually no one believed exercise would help a person to lose weight. Until the 1960s, clinicians who treated obese and overweight persons dismissed the notion as naive. When Russell Wilder, an obesity and diabetes specialist at the Mayo Clinic, lectured on obesity in 1932, he said his fat patients tended to lose more weight with bed rest, "while unusually strenuous exercise slows down the rate of loss" (Taube, 2007, p 2). But the most obvious question that needs to be answered is whether people are actually doing less physical exercise now than they used to. This is difficult to determine retrospectively, but according to the General Household Survey 2002, 75% of adults in the UK claimed to have taken part in a sport, game or physical activity in the 12 months before interview, while participation in sports had increased overall since 1987. While these data are not necessarily reliable, they do not suggest an inexorable decrease in physical activity. However, Morris (1995) quotes UK Sports Council data that appear to show that "participation [in activity] is increasing across all age bands and all social groupings". The picture seems to be similar in the US, for instance Pratt et al (1999) suggest that instead of a decline, "levels of physical activity and inactivity as measured by the BRFSS and NIS have been remarkably stable"(p 6).The case for increasing sedentariness is not quite so easy to argue as it might seem. In addition, there is scarce evidence to link lack of exercise to obesity and health. As Sobal and Stunkard (1989) point out:

> A major problem in population studies ... is the apparent lack of relationship between food intake, physical exercise and body weight of adults (Keen et al, 1979; Keen et al, 1982; Kromhout, 1983), adolescents (Bingham et al, 1981; Hampton et al, 1967) and infants (Vobecky et al, 1983).

Given that the link between obesity and lack of exercise is taken for granted there is a lack of evidence to conclusively demonstrate the relationship. Hill and Melanson (1999) state that "while the amount of physical activity that protects against obesity is not known there is however, plenty of 'indirect' evidence to suggest that this is the case". Indirect evidence refers to longitudinal population studies, which rely heavily upon self-reported data and can only offer co-relational, not causal conclusions about the relationship between physical activity and body weight (Gard and Wright, 2005). Grundy et al (1999) and Wing (1999) have shown that studies which add exercise alone to an individual's life-style have produced very modest or, in some cases, no weight reduction. Numerous studies show that the relationship between body weight and physical activity is inconsistent, unclear or controversial. The extent to which exercise contributes to weight (or fat) loss is regularly described in the literature as small, disappointing or modest (Ballor and Keensey, 1991; Robinson, 1999), or even non-existent (Shephard, 1997). For example, Taube (2007) refers to a report that he claims is "the most scientifically rigorous review of the evidence to date" (p 3) and which concludes that the link between physical activity and obesity is "more complex" than scientists had thought. Taube also offers anecdotal evidence from Steve Blair, a University of South Carolina exercise scientist who "was short, fat and bald when he started running in his thirties and he is short, fatter and balder now at the age of 68. In the intervening years he estimates he has run close to 80,000 miles and gained about 30lb" (p 2).

Another complicating factor in the debate concerns the intensity of exercise, as opposed to the amount. While a number of studies (Pollock, 1992; LeMura and Maziekas, 2002) have been conducted, none seems to be able to answer this deceptively simple question convincingly in the case of adults, and a similar confusion remains when considering childhood obesity (Wolf et al, 1993; Fogelholm et al, 1999; Grund et al, 2001; Schutz and Mafeis, 2002). For example, after reviewing the literature, Sleap et al (2000) concluded that the evidence that childhood health and obesity are related to physical activity is difficult to find. Boreham and Riddoch (2003) reached a similar conclusion. They write:

> Although we feel instinctively that physical activity ought to be beneficial to the health of children, there is surprisingly little empirical evidence to support this notion. (p 17)

Nonetheless, this link is endlessly pursued in the media and literature. The alleged generation of couch potatoes is accused of watching too much television, playing too many computer games and not doing enough sport. The couch potato accusation is also not universally supported by empirical evidence. Grund et al (2001) found that the link between watching television and childhood obesity is inconsistent, and Wake et al (2003) reported similar findings in their study of 5- to 13-year-olds. Similarly, the link between sports and childhood obesity is so frequently reported that it has achieved the status of truth. This is sometimes linked into the debate around the idea that, in terms of sporting activity, "we ain't the way we used to be". Gard and Wright (2005) point out that child health and the obesity epidemic are often used as grounds for objecting to the sale of school playing fields. They point to Sian Griffith's 2002 *Sunday Times* article 'Heading for the top', in which she makes connections between a whole range of assumptions, issues and problems without explaining what evidence there is to support any of them. They comment that what is implied is that:

> high academic achievement is the same as 'having a healthy mind', that physical exercise not only leads to a 'healthy mind' but also 'good behaviour' and 'self discipline', that boys need and are more inclined towards physical activity than girls, that sport is 'healthy'. These assumptions are not so much 'facts' as part of an ideology which supports a diverse list of social and moral domains. (Gard and Wright, 2005, p 30)

Obesity: the result of eating too much?

The link with physical activity is unclear, and the link between eating too much and obesity is also surprisingly complicated. Generally speaking, there is a shared understanding that obesity is caused by consuming more calories than are expended. This model is used by Foresight and other government agencies and is relied upon in most scientific and lay discussions of obesity. However, this relies on the assumption that the body is like a machine that functions with predictable mechanics. As Gard and Wright comment:

> Whether or not excessive food intake causes overweight and obesity is controversial. The idea that overeating causes fatness has a long history and yet it is an idea which researchers are still trying to prove. (2005, p 45)

The premise that obesity is directly related to excessive calorie intake (especially saturated fat intake) is rarely questioned in health promotion literature. Yet researchers have been questioning the relationship for years. Writing more than 20 years ago, Wooley and Wooley (1984) advanced the idea that the relationship between overeating and obesity was not as straightforward as suggested, and they noted that it was possible for some people to maintain a high body weight on very few calories. In addition there is the conundrum that with unrelenting healthy eating campaigns being run by GPs, public health professionals and the media, people are consuming fewer calories and less saturated fat than ever before (Salbe and Ravussin, 2000; Willett and Leibel, 2002), and yet we are facing an obesity epidemic. Furthermore, research that has studied the effect on body weight of restricting calories consistently shows that it is not very effective, and that individuals who succeed in reducing their body weight regain at least the same amount of weight when the programme finishes, and often gain significantly more (Stunkard and Penrick, 1979; Frank, 1993; Robinson, 1999; Stice et al, 1999; Swinburn and Egger, 2002; Field et al, 2003).

Is being overweight unhealthy?

What the above discussion clearly shows is that 'what everyone knows' about the causes of overweight and obesity may not be correct. But does it really matter if we have not got the causes of the obesity epidemic nailed down? Which brings us to the well-known concept that being overweight or obese is unhealthy. Part of this debate revolves around whether or not obesity is in itself a disease or a risk factor for other diseases. This chapter concentrates on the latter.

The idea that obesity is a risk factor for other diseases is another example of something 'everyone knows', with non-insulin dependent diabetes and heart disease perhaps being the two most commonly cited. However, designing studies to confirm this association is difficult and tends to conflate incidence and prevalence. As Ross (2005) points out:

> It is difficult to design epidemiological studies that follow a cohort of people long enough and in enough detail to show a clear relationship between the incidence of a disease and the incidence of obesity. Most studies report the prevalence, not the incidence of obesity in a population, and relate that to the incidence of various diseases over relatively short periods of time. Alternatively, they compare the prevalence of obesity and the incidence of disease with a comparable cohort years later. Thus at best, the data suggests a correlation between obesity prevalence and disease incidence. (p 88)

In other words, the data do not establish a cause-and-effect relationship. Indeed, it has been claimed that there is no justification at all in saying that obesity causes ischaemic heart disease or non-insulin dependent diabetes (Bradford Hill, 1977; Skrabanek, 1992; Krieger, 1994; Pearce, 1996). Ross (2005) also points out that obesity could actually be a symptom of non-insulin dependent diabetes rather than a cause. An alternative explanation for the rise in non-insulin dependent diabetes in America is offered by Ernsberger:

> the definition of diabetes was changed from a fasting blood sugar level of 140 to a blood sugar level of 126. Thus millions of Americans became diabetic overnight, we are also an aging population, and diabetes rises exponentially after the age of 50. (Cited in Campos, 2004, p 22)

Campos has claimed that being overweight can protect against certain serious conditions such as hip fracture and chronic obstructive pulmonary disease, among others. All of which raises the question why, if the evidence that overweight and obesity is so equivocal, we are urged to diet, exercise and remain a 'healthy' weight.

Money and weight

GPs in the UK are under increasing pressure to monitor patients on an opportunity basis and record those whose BMI is higher than 25, even though BMI is well known to be a poor measure of human adiposity, as is the alternative of using the measurement of waist and hip circumference (Wooley and Wooley, 1984; Flegal et al, 2002; Boreham and Riddoch, 2003). Not only is BMI an insensitive measure, but it does not take into account the diversity of male and female physique, let alone ethnic differences (Prentice and Jebb, 2001). The Quality Outcomes Framework of the new General Medical Services contract incorporates points for registering patients aged 16 and over with a BMI higher than 25 – a voluntary requirement completed by all practices, for which they receive payment. From an ethical perspective, medical pressure on patients might possibly be justified if it at least *did no harm*; however, this chapter does not contend this. What is happening is that fatness is becoming increasingly stigmatised as 'scientific' health information is incorporated into a pre-existing set of cultural beliefs that fat people are either gluttonous or slothful (or both), and that their lack of self-control and moral fibre is costing millions of pounds every year in medical treatment and lost earnings. This is constantly reinforced by the so-called 'diet industry' and by media messages which clearly tell us that to be slim is good and desirable. These are messages that seem to be equally acceptable across the political spectrum. It has been estimated that the global weight-loss market is in the region of $240 billion, and Campos (2004) has calculated that in the US approximately 70 million adults are dieting to lose weight, and another 45 million are dieting to maintain their weight at any given time. There is little evidence that the quest for a slimmer body will necessarily lead to a healthier body. Indeed, individuals who do manage to lose weight on diets almost always regain it, and frequently gain more than they originally lost. Moreover, some have suggested that repeated weight loss and gain is detrimental to health. For example, Gaesser (2002) states:

> If a hypertensive obese person follows the advice to lose weight in order to lower blood pressure and the remedy doesn't work (as it often doesn't), then what you have is a weight reduced hypertensive who is now statistically more likely to die from cardiovascular disease than before. (Cited in Campos, 2004, p 21)

Repeated weight loss and gain has been shown in a number of studies to be unhealthy, and yet individuals who are even moderately fat are made to feel that they are medically at risk. However, while overweight and obesity have been increasingly medicalised, the social and cultural effects of the discourse around the ideal body also have important consequences. Twigg (2006) comments that "fat has come to be evaluated negatively in terms of sexual attractiveness, slothfulness and low social class" (p 103).

This particularly affects women in the developed world, where they are constantly bombarded with images of the perfect body, and the resulting dissatisfaction with their own bodies is well documented. Bordo (2004) adds that as slenderness is "glamorised", any "softness or bulge comes to be seen as unsightly – as disgusting, disorderly fat which must be eliminated or busted, as popular exercise equipment ads put it" (p 97). Not only must the female body be slim to conform to the ideal, but it must now also be taut and muscular. Howell and Ingham (2001) point out:

> For women, health and physical attractiveness were conflated in the appearance of the body. Social norms not only required a thin body but also evidence of a worked body. (p 33)

While some have argued that there has been a move to be happy with your body whatever its size, Bordo argues that this too has become incorporated into the 'ideal':

> The mythology persists, of course ... Jenifer Lopez and Beyonce Knowles insist that they are happy with their bodies – bragging about their bodacious bottoms ... but sexy booty is okay, apparently, only if its high and hard and if other body parts are held firmly in check ... Beyonce is 'happy with her body' because she works on it ... on the road she does five hundred sit ups a night and ninety minutes of hard training at least four times a week. (2004, p xxii)

Bordo (2004), among others (Chernin, 1981), has argued that the current obsession with slenderness has led to an unprecedented rise in eating disorders. The idea that an individual can diet and exercise their way to a better body has turned out to be something of an empty promise which has led some to a lifetime of weight-related misery and guilt. Campos (2004) interviewed 400 people with regard to their struggle with overweight, and the one interview reproduced here is a typical experience:

> In the days when I did diet, I tried just about every one out there, at one time or another. Atkins, fasting pills, Simmons,

grapefruit, carb addicts, medically issued amphetamines and diuretics, lots of fruits and veggies, broiled meat, no meat, Lean Cuisine: I'm sure there are few, if any that I didn't try over a thirty year time span. Talk about self abuse! I spent the majority of my life trapped inside that insane cycle.... the result of dieting most of my life was years of wasted energy, misery, and a sense of being an unmitigated failure, because no matter how hard I tried, how much I brutalised myself, I could never accomplish what the 'establishment' said I would if I just showed some 'self discipline'. Damn them all. They should have half the 'discipline' I imposed on myself in all those.

Caught between a food industry which is attempting to seduce people into eating more (major supermarkets, such as Tesco, continue to advertise their food range, and particularly chocolate, specifically aimed at women) and the increasing range of low-fat, fat-free, diet and low-calorie foods with names like 'Go Ahead', not to mention the over-the-counter (and under-the-counter) medicines which promise weight loss – at a price – and the increasing medicalised stigmatisation of overweight and obese people, it is hardly surprising that we, as a society, are developing a very uneasy relationship with both our bodies and the food we eat. As 'consumers' we are being encouraged to 'eat ourselves thin and healthy' by eating more nutritionally dodgy foods, while being told by the advertisers that we are 'protecting our heart' or that by eating their products we will be not only healthy but happy. In addition, this needs to be placed into a context where people are getting generally larger. To take a very long historical context, Wilford (1997) points out that:

> The celebrated Lucy, a fossil female from 3.2 million years ago, was a diminutive adult, 3 feet 7 inches tall and no more than 60 pounds. Another skeleton found in related African fossil beds, presumably that of a male, measured 5 feet 3 inches and 110 pounds.

There is evidence that the difference in sizes (dimorphism) between men and women is decreasing. In many primate species, males are 35%–40% larger than females, and for Neanderthal humans, males were 35% larger than females. This difference has declined steadily, and modern males are approximately 15% larger than females. This resonates with more recent evidence. The biggest women's clothing retailer in the UK (Marks and Spencer) recently measured thousands of women and compared the results with its archives, which date back to the 1920s. The results show that in the UK, the average woman's bust has grown by four inches and gone from a B to a C cup. Her waist is eight inches bigger. Six inches have been added to her hips. She is one inch taller and her feet are up to two sizes larger. Overall, the average 32B-20-32 (measured in inches) figure of the 1920s has been replaced by 36C-28-38 today. This is interesting from a sociological point of view, for as the physical size of the average woman has increased, the desirability of slenderness has made the 'ideal' female body shape more difficult to attain, with the potential for causing more misery, stress and psychosocial repercussions for both men and women.

Implications for practice

In the 'war against obesity', health professionals are increasingly required to measure and monitor people, and where someone's BMI is considered too high, to take remedial action. In the UK, the government has declared 'war on obesity' (Hynde, 2008), echoing the US war on obesity launched several years ago, which has tended to be a war on the obese rather than on obesity (Campos et al, 2006). However, concerns remain as to whether such an approach will bring results (Friedman, 2003; Waine, 2007). More importantly, the characterisation of tackling obesity as a war may also have negative consequences by stigmatising particular groups in the population (Saguy and Riley, 2005).

The focus on obesity presents it as a disease, raising the question of whether the medical profession has been seduced into a campaign of surveillance of BMI in the mistaken belief that obesity is a 'disease' in itself, rather than a risk factor for other diseases. Yet, as has been demonstrated in this chapter, the link between obesity and these other diseases is not clear. Studies show a correlation rather than a cause-and-effect relationship. Recent recommendations by doctors that more bariatric surgery should be conducted on people with lower BMI than is currently recommended, in order to reduce diabetes and other symptoms of obesity (Randerson, 2008), demonstrate the metamorphosis of being overweight into a disease to be addressed by medical intervention. Current NICE guidelines restrict surgery to people with a BMI of 40 kg/m^2 or more, or between 35 kg/m^2 and 40 kg/m^2 and other significant disease (for example, Type 2 diabetes or high blood pressure) that could be improved if they lost weight and where other non-surgical measures have failed. Thus, the suggestion that even those with a BMI of 25 or over should be eligible for surgery demonstrates the increasing medicalisation of the body and medical surveillance of behaviour. This raises important questions about what approaches are prioritised for supporting people who want to reduce their weight and whether the desire to lose weight is primarily driven by social and medical pressure.

This medicalisation of obesity represents a new version of Calvinism – one that the medical profession appears to support – where restraint and control (over behaviour/consumption) have become a central plank in the new public health. This is ethically highly dubious, as the general public are led to believe that all they need to do is diet and exercise, and the golden chalice of good health will be theirs.

If medicine is to be 'evidence based', then public health practitioners need to be more rigorous that what becomes the accepted wisdom is indeed 'evidence' and not simply an irresistible force based on assumption as well as on moral and ideological beliefs. Increasing standardisation of what constitutes being overweight or obese, and of how this is measured and dealt with by health professionals, also raises the issue of choice and freedom for individuals. Are people to be cajoled and medicated simply because they are deemed to fall into a risk category, even if they themselves are not at risk from any specific health problem, or because their risk of a disease is 'potentially higher'? As Campos et al (2006) argue:

> Except at true statistical extremes, high body mass is a very weak predictor of mortality, and may even be protective in older populations. In particular, the claim that 'overweight' (BMI 25–29.9) increases mortality risk in any meaningful way is impossible to reconcile with numerous large-scale studies that have found no increase in relative risk among the so-called 'overweight', or have found a lower relative risk for premature mortality among this cohort than among persons of so-called 'normal' or 'ideal' weight. (p 56)

In the UK, as in the US, it appears that it is 'common knowledge' (or perhaps mis-knowledge) that appears to be framing health policy on obesity. The labelling of people as obese and requiring medical intervention is founded on value-based rather than evidence-based approaches. Health professionals are also increasingly drawn into routine surveillance of people's bodies and lives, perhaps reinforcing particular sets of values about the nature of obesity.

Note
[1] There are clearly issues regarding the definitions of overweight and obesity, but for the purposes of this chapter it is assumed that 'obesity' and 'overweight' are unproblematic categories. We acknowledge that this is not the case.

References

Ballor, D.L. and Keensey, R.E. (1991) 'A meta analysis of the factors affecting exercise-induced changes in body mass, fat mass and fat-free mass in males and females', *International Journal of Obesity*, vol 15, no 11, pp 717–26.

Bordo, S. (2004) *Unbearable weight*, London: University of California Press.

Boreham, C. and Riddoch, C. (2003) 'Physical activity and health through the lifespan', in J. McKenna and C. Riddoch (eds) *Perspectives on health and exercise*, Basingstoke: Palgrave.

Bradford Hill, A. (1977) *A short textbook of medical statistics*, London: Hodder and Stoughton.

Campos, J.D., Saguy, A., Ernsberger, P., Oliver, E. and Gaesser, G. (2006) 'The epidemiology of overweight and obesity: public health crisis or moral panic?', *International Journal of Epidemiology*, vol 35, no 1, pp 55–60.

Campos, P. (2004) *The obesity myth: Why America's obsession with weight is hazardous to your health*, New York: Gotham Books.

Chernin, K. (1981) *The hungry self: Women, eating and identity*, New York: Harper Paperbacks.

DH (Department of Health) (2008) *Healthy weight, healthy lives: A cross-government strategy for England*, London: Department of Health. Available at: www.dh.gov.uk/en/Publicationsandstatistics/Publications/PublicationsPolicyAndGuidance/DH_082378 (accessed 24 September 2008).

Ells, L.J., Macknight, N. and Williamson, J.R. (2007) 'Obesity surgery in England: an examination of the health episode statistics 1996–2005', *Obesity Surgery*, vol 17, no 3, pp 400–5.

Field, A.E., Austin, S.B., Taylor, C.B., Malspecis, S., Rosner, B., Rockett, H.R., Gillman, M.W. and Colditz, G.A. (2003) 'Relation between dieting and weight change among pre-adolescents and adolescents', *Paediatrics*, vol 112, no 4, pp 900–6.

Flegal, K.M., Carroll, M.D., Ogden, C.L. and Johnson, C.L. (2002) 'Prevalence and trends in obesity among US adults, 1999–2000', *Journal of the American Medical Association*, vol 288, no 14, pp 1772–3.

Fogelholm, M., Nuutinen, O., Pasanen, M., Myohanen, E. and Saatela, T. (1999) 'Parent- –child relationship of physical activity patterns and obesity', *International Journal of Obesity and Related Metabolic Disorders*, vol 23, no 12, pp 1262–8.

Frank, A. (1993) 'Futility and avoidance: medical professionals in the treatment of obesity', *Journal of the American Medical Association*, vol 269, no 16, pp 2132–3.

Friedman, J.M. (2003) 'A war on obesity not the obese', *Science*, vol 299, no 5608, pp 856–8.

Gaesser, G. (2002) *Big fat lies: The truth about your weight and your health*, Carlsbad, CA: Gurze Books.

Gard, M. and Wright, J. (eds) (2005) *The obesity epidemic: Science, morality and ideology*, Abingdon: Routledge.

Goldstein, M.S. (1992) *The health movement: Promoting fitness in America*, New York: Twayne Publishers.

Government Office for Science (2007) *ForeSight: Modelling future trends in obesity and the impact on health*. Available at: www.foresight.gov.uk/index.aspl (accessed 24 September 2008).

Griffiths, S. (2002) 'Heading for the top', *Sunday Times*, 10 March.

Grund, A., Krause, H., Siewers, M., Rieckert, H. and Muller, M.J. (2001) 'Is TV viewing an index of physical activity and fitness in overweight and normal weight children?' *Public Health Nutrition*, vol 4, no 6, pp 1245–51.

Grundy, S.M., Blackburn, G., Higgins, M., Lauer, R., Perri, M. and Ryan, D. (1999) 'Physical activity in the prevention and treatment of obesity and its comorbidities', *Medicine and Science in Sports and Exercise*, vol 31, no 11 (suppl), s502–8.

Hill, J. and Melanson, E.L. (1999) 'Overview of the determinants of overweight and obesity: current evidence and research issues', *Medicine and Science in Sports and Exercise*, vol 31, no 11 (suppl), s515–21.

House of Commons Health Select Committee (2004) *Obesity, Third Report Session 2003–04*, HC 23-I, London: House of Commons.

Howell, J. and Ingham, A. (2001) 'From social problem to personal issue: the language of lifestyle', *Cultural Studies*, vol 15, no 2, pp 326–51.

Hynde, M. (2008) 'The war on obesity must be won round the cabinet table', *Guardian*, 26 January.

Krieger, N. (1994) 'Epidemiology and the web of causation: has anyone seen the spider?', *Social Science and Medicine*, vol 39, no 7, pp 887–903.

LeMura, L. and Maziekas, M.T. (2002) 'Factors that alter body fat, body mass and fat-free mass in pediatric obesity', *Medicine in Science and Sports and Exercise*, vol 34, no 3, pp 487–96.

Lichtarowitz, A. (2007) 'Obesity "out of control"', *BBC World Service*. Available at http://news.bbc.co.uk/nolpda/ukfs/hi/newsid_3969000/3969693.stm (accessed 8 July 2008).

Morris, J.N. (1995) 'Obesity in Britain: lifestyle data do not support sloth hypothesis', *British Medical Journal*, vol 311, no 7002, pp 437–9.

NHS (2006) *Statistics on obesity, physical activity and diet: England, 2006.* Available at www.ic.nhs.uk/statistics-and-data-collections/health-and-lifestyles/obesity/statistics-on-obesity-physical-activity-and-diet-england-2006 (accessed 16 September 2008).

NICE (2008) *Obesity guidelines*, CG 43, London: NICE.

Pearce, N. (1996) 'Traditional epidemiology, modern epidemiology, and public health', *American Journal of Public Health*, vol 86, no 5, pp 678–83.

Pollock, C.L. (1992) 'Does exercise intensity matter?', *Physician and Sports Medicine*, vol 20, no 12, pp 123–6.

Pratt, M., Macera, C.A. and Blanton, C. (1999) 'Levels of physical activity and inactivity in children and adults in the United States: current evidence and research issues', *Medicine and Science in Sports and Exercise*, vol 31, no 11 (suppl), s526–33.

Prentice, A.M. and Jebb, S.A. (2001) 'Beyond body mass index', *Obesity Reviews*, vol 2, no 3, pp 141–7.

Randerson, J. (2008) 'Scientists call for huge increase in gastric bypass surgery to tackle obesity crisis', *Guardian*, 8 September.

Robinson, T.N. (1999) 'Reducing children's television viewing to prevent obesity: a randomised controlled trial', *Journal of the American Medical Association*, vol 282, no 16, pp 1561–7.

Ross, B. (2005) 'Fat or fiction: weighing the "obesity epidemic"', in M. Gard and J. Wright (eds) *The obesity epidemic: Science, morality and ideology*, London: Routledge, pp 86–106.

Saguy, A.C. and Riley, K.W. (2005) 'Weighing both sides: morality, mortality and framing contests over obesity', *Journal of Health Politics, Policy and Law*, vol 30, no 5, pp 869–921.

Salbe, A.D. and Ravussin, E. (2000) 'The determinants of obesity', in C. Bouchlard (ed) *Physical activity and obesity*, Champaign, IL: Human Kinetics.

Schutz, Y. and Mafeis, C. (2002) 'Physical activity', in W. Burniat, T. Cole, L. Lissay and E. Poskitt (eds) *Child and adolescent obesity: Causes and consequences, prevention and management*, Cambridge: Cambridge University Press.

Shephard, R.J. (1997) 'What is the optimal type of physical activity to enhance health?', *International Journal of Sports Medicine*, vol 87, no 5, pp 615–9.

Sleap, M., Warburton, P. and Waring, M. (2000) 'Couch potato kids and lazy layabouts: the role of primary schools in relation to physical activity among children', in A. Williams (ed) *Primary schools physical education: Research into practice*, Lewes: Routledge.

Skrabanek, P. (1992) 'The poverty of epidemiology', *Perspectives in Biology and Medicine*, vol 35, no 2, pp 182–5.

Sobal, J. and Stunkard, A. (1989) 'The socioeconomic status and obesity: a review of the literature', *Psychological Bulletin*, vol 105, no 2, pp 260–75.

Stice, E., Cameron, R.P., Killen, J.D., Hayward, C. and Taylor, C.B. (1999) 'Naturalistic weight reduction efforts prospectively predict growth in relative weight and onset of obesity among female adolescents', *Journal of Consulting and Clinical Psychology*, vol 67, no 6, pp 967–74.

Stunkard, A.J. and Penick, S.B. (1979) 'Behaviour modification in the treatment of obesity – the problems of maintaining health loss', *Archives of General Psychiatry*, vol 36, no 7, pp 801–6.

Swinburn, B. and Egger, G. (2002) 'Preventive strategies against weight gain and obesity', *Obesity Reviews*, vol 3, no 2, pp 289–301.

Taube, G. (2007) 'We can't work it out', *Observer*, 28 October.

Twigg, J. (2006) 'The body in health and social care', London: Palgrave Macmillan.

Waine, C. (2007) 'Shame game "losing" war on obesity', *Scotland on Sunday*, 22 July.

Wake, K., Hesketh, K. and Waters, E. (2003) 'Television, computer use and BMI in Australian primary school children', *Journal of Paediatrics and Child Health*, vol 39, no 2, pp 130–4.

Wanless, D. (2004) *Securing good health for the whole population*, London: HM Treasury.

Wilford, J.N. (1997) 'New clues to history of male and female', *New York Times*, 26 August. Available at: http://query.nytimes.com/gst/fullpage.html?res=9F05E3DD1F3EF935A1575BC0A961958260&sec=&spon=&pagewanted=2 (accessed 24 September 2008).

Willett, W.C. and Leibel, R.L. (2002) 'Is dietary fat a major determinant of body fat?', *American Journal of Clinical Nutrition*, vol 113, no 9B (suppl), pp 47–59.

Wing, R.R. (1999) 'Physical activity in the treatment of adult overweight and obesity: current evidence and research issues', *Medicine and Science in Sport and Exercise*, vol 31, no 11 (suppl), s547–52.

Wolf, A.M., Gortmaker, S.L., Cheung, L., Gray, H.M., Herzog, D.B. and Colditz, G.A. (1993) 'Activity, inactivity and obesity: racial, ethnic and age differences among schoolgirls', *American Journal of Public Health*, vol 83, no 11, pp 1625–7.

Wooley, S.C. and Wooley, O.W. (1984) 'Should obesity be treated at all?', in A.J. Stunkard and E. Stellar (eds) *Eating and its disorders*, New York: Raven Press.

World Health Organization (2007) 'WHO Global infobase online', Geneva: World Health Organization. Available at: www.who.int/infobase/report.aspx (accessed 24 September 2008).

World Health Organization (2008) 'Controlling the global obesity epidemic', Geneva: World Health Organization. Available at: www.who.int/nutrition/topics/obesity/en/print.html (accessed 8 July 2008).

NINE

Politics, ethics and evidence: immunisation and public health policy

Alison Hann and Stephen Peckham

This chapter explores the relationship between ethics and practice and the basis upon which public health interventions can be applied. The justification for vaccination programmes is based on differing values and principles and therefore vaccination requires an exploration of ethical approaches. The chapter explores what kinds of ethical approaches public health practitioners can adopt in support of developing and implementing public health programmes. This has been a recurrent theme in this book and the area of immunisation is a particularly useful one to explore in this context.

Introduction

Public health interventions are rarely without harmful as well as beneficial effect. As Kenny and Giacomini (2005) argue:

> when many people – as well as societal constructs such as institutions and economies – are affected in many ways by every decision, the moral quandaries arise not in the question of *whether* to harm or benefit but *how* to harm *and* benefit: whom, how much, how certainly, in what ways, and so forth ... The quintessential ethical problem of the public policy maker is how to define, identify, justify, and distribute inevitable benefits and harms, rather than simply striving to ensure benefit and avoid harm. (p 254)

This is a well-recognised dilemma in all public policy, but public health raises important questions about not only the degree or distribution of harm or benefit but also how to define those harms and benefits. For example, a key debate in public health is the extent to which it is right to intervene to restrict a person's liberty to protect them and/or others from harm. In addition policy makers may formulate policy that needs to *look* good, not necessarily *be* good for purely self-interested political goals, or because seeming to do something is seen as promoting the greatest benefit.

In this chapter we examine some of these issues, using vaccination programmes as a case study. It is not our intention to question the benefit or otherwise of any particular vaccination programme or to argue that any specific programme is right or wrong, but rather to use the example of vaccination to explore public health ethics and to examine the link between ethics, evidence and public health policy.

There is a huge investment in vaccination programmes in the UK and worldwide as a preventive public health measure to improve population health. However, vaccination remains a controversial issue and the subject of media and political debate, such as the continuing furore around the MMR vaccine. In addition, changes in policy are difficult to justify and implement, as immunisation is seen to confer population benefit, and thus suggestions to change dosage and frequency or to stop programmes mean a perception that benefit will be reduced. Similarly, the introduction of new vaccines raises important ethical questions relating to how evidence is obtained and clinical and population safety are verified.

Governments and public health professionals continue to justify the programmes as being both medically and ethically good, as the evidence supporting population vaccination is strong, with benefits far outweighing any potential harm. Policy is based on the need to maintain 'herd immunity', to confer population benefit. Put very simply, herd immunity is the notion that "If enough people in the community are immunised, the infection can no longer be spread from person to person and the disease dies out altogether" (WHO, 2005). Thus, vaccination represents a classic case of a social dilemma: a potential conflict of interests between the private gains of individuals and the collective gains of a society. In this country, the choice to vaccinate is based on an individual's free choice (although this is heavily influenced by orthodox medical evidence and social norms; see below), and it is important to note at this point that the individual's choice is based on imperfect information and that the vaccination choice involves a positive externality.[1] However, people make choices based on their calculation of *individual* gains (and costs), without taking into consideration the social impact of their decisions. People choosing not to vaccinate are seen as being beneficiaries (or a kind of free rider)[2] of herd immunity, and are subjected to social disapproval. Those parents who choose not to vaccinate their children (for example) are vilified in the press or are accused by health professionals of putting their and other children at risk (Jansen et al, 2003). Questions of autonomy and parental choice and control have been tested in court where divorced parents have disagreed about the immunisation of their child. In one case the judge ruled against the wishes of both the mother and the child (who at the time was aged 10), claiming that the mother had a 'unreasoning and rigid approach' and that he could therefore 'discount her concerns' over the safety of the combined MMR vaccine (*Guardian*, 2001). To maintain high immunisation rates and 'herd immunity', the government and health services actively promote vaccination and, while it is voluntary in the UK, employ routine procedures and standardisation of vaccination programmes, including patient recall systems (GP targets), publicity campaigns and school-based delivery programmes to ensure maximum coverage – sometimes in the face of growing evidence questioning the efficacy of programmes. For example, until 2007 the BCG vaccination programme was actively promoted in secondary schools, despite questions about the efficacy of the programme, which had been questioned for a number of years – finally leading to its withdrawal. Does this make the policy to promote BCG vaccination in the first place a bad policy? This returns us to the dilemma mentioned earlier. Given that the social benefit of vaccination programmes rests on herd immunity, and that this can only be achieved if a high percentage of the population at risk gets the vaccine, should the choice be left to the individual? This begs the question of the extent to which the state should coerce citizens into being vaccinated – especially if this coercion is based on imperfect information.[3] This raises important ethical questions.

The ethical dimension

What do we mean by ethical? Typically, a moral or ethical statement asserts that some particular action is right or wrong, or that certain kinds of action are right or wrong, or it may propose some kind of general principle from which we might determine which actions are right and which are wrong. For example, we may have the principle that we must always try to aim for the greatest general happiness, or try to minimise the total suffering of all human beings (sometimes expressed as 'all those concerned'); or perhaps we should devote ourselves completely to the service and worship of God, or we must try to do what is dutiful and fulfil our obligations to others; or perhaps it's a case of 'every man [*sic*] for himself'. Now, whichever approach might be taken, it would seem self-evident that any public health measure that conferred only good outcomes (such as clean drinking water) must be 'ethical' (provided that in doing so no one was harmed or had their rights violated). Sadly, few public health measures are so cut and dried. In the case of vaccination programmes, it is known that certain vaccinations may damage or cause harm to some individuals, and while most of these harmful effects are considered minor, some effects of vaccination lead to more serious complications. For example, the data sheet produced by the manufacturer for M-M-R 11 (Merck Sharpe and Dohme, 2006) lists under 'Adverse Effects' symptoms which range from "Burning and/or stinging of short duration at the injection site" (p 6) to "convulsions" and "death" (p 6). Thus, the calculation of whether a vaccination programme is 'good' or not involves some kind of balance between the benefits and harms. This is further complicated by sometimes conflicting medical evidence, individual freedom of choice, societal benefits, and the right of the state to enforce compliance, and to what degree.

One argument for population immunisation is based on the utilitarian premise that an action is right if and only if it promotes the best consequences for the largest number of people. This approach is eloquently summarised by Spock in *Star Trek: The Motion Picture* as "the needs of the many outweigh the needs of the few". This provides a specification of right action, making the link between 'rightness' and best consequences, but this, in itself, doesn't give any real guidance on what counts as a 'best consequence'. Thus, a second premise is required in that the best consequences are those in which happiness (or utility) is maximised. So we might modify Spock's formulation to "the happiness (utility) of the many outweighs the happiness (utility) of the few".[4]

Utilitarianism has a long and illustrious pedigree, having gone through numerous permutations in the hands of philosophers, economists and politicians who have been attracted to its potential for social reform (Oliver, 2006). Its roots can be found in trying to understand human behaviour and Aristotelian ideas about human flourishing (or eudemonics), but has since evolved into terms such as preference satisfaction or utility (Mill, 1974). Thus, where an agent has a choice between courses of action (or inaction), the right act is the one that will produce the most 'utility', usually understood as benefit or happiness. To achieve this, it is necessary to be able to add up all the amounts of utility it produces for all who are in 'any way affected', and similarly to add up and measure all the amounts of pain (harm/misery) the action produces, and then subtract the amount of pain from the amount of harm. The right action will then be the one for which there is the greatest positive (or the least negative) balance. This has several obvious attractions. It would seem reasonable that morality, if it is going to guide conduct, should have something to do with happiness, flourishing or benefit. It would also seem natural to seek to avoid pain or harm, and also to balance the one against the other. In taking the *general* happiness or benefit as a standard of right action, utilitarianism seems to satisfy the presumption that moral actions should be unselfish and fair (Mackie, 1977). This balancing of benefits and harm would seem ideally suited, at first consideration, to public health interventions, vaccination being an eminently suitable case in point. Balance the misery and death caused by, say, smallpox or polio against the relatively small risks and side effects of the vaccination, and it would seem that vaccinating for smallpox must be a right action, as defined above. However, what about vaccination for rarer diseases, or those creating fewer complications, such as chickenpox, influenza or hepatitis B? However, before we deal with the specific problems raised by particular public health interventions, we need to consider some of the standard problems raised by utilitarianism, or its specific interpretation here of act utilitarianism (Mackie, 1977).

The difficulties are well known and have been well rehearsed elsewhere, so we will mention them here only briefly. First, what are we to include in 'all who are in any way affected'? Does this mean all human beings or all sentient beings? Does it include those who are now alive, or also future generations? Is it really possible to measure harm and benefit in the way required by act utilitarianism? For example, supposing vaccination greatly benefited 20% of the people, and was only mildly unpleasant for 55%, while 15% were caused long-term and severe suffering. A classic utilitarian might well judge that this was a good trade-off, but how we identify benefit and harm and the degree of benefit or harm is also clearly important in making such an assessment. Further difficulties are also raised by the recognition that act utilitarianism focuses primarily on the outcome and not on the means to achieve it. Thus, it would be possible to tolerate the use of torture or violence if this leads to the maximisation of the general good. Thus, utilitarianism not only allows, but enjoins, in some circumstances, that the benefit (utility) of 'the many' might be 'purchased' at the cost of the undeserved and uncompensated misery of 'the few'. This raises questions of rights and justice which Mill himself recognised, and which have been extensively discussed in the literature (Mackie, 1977; Kymlicka, 1990).

There is also a difficulty when it comes to weighing the distribution of harm and utility within the life of any individual. A period of misery followed by one of happiness seems preferable to a period of happiness followed by one of misery, even if the *quantities* are equal. In addition, are we talking about *expected* utility or *actual* utility? Clearly, we do not always have perfect information concerning all the possible outcomes of actions. And lastly, there is no specification in utilitarianism that certain acts are 'immoral' even if they do promote the greatest benefit. For example there is no requirement to always tell the truth, be compassionate, keep promises or be loyal. So, for example, if the kind of utility that is being maximised is, say, freedom from worry or distress, then a lie – if it maximises this – is preferable to the truth.

One attempt at dealing with these problems is to introduce moral rules (rule utilitarianism). This holds that the rightness of an action is *not* to be tested simply by evaluating its consequences, but by considering whether it falls under a certain rule. Whether the rule is to be considered an acceptable moral rule is, however, decided by considering the consequences of adopting that rule. As Kymlicka explains it: "we should apply the test of utility to rules, and then perform whichever act is endorsed by the rules, even if another act might produce more utility. Social co-operation requires rule-following, so we should assess the consequences, not simply of acting in a particular way on this occasion, but of making it a rule that we act in that way" (1990, p 27). However, rule utilitarianism also has a fatal flaw. Sometimes, in order to act morally we need to make exceptions to rules – especially when rules come into conflict. In order to take account of this, the rule utilitarian may wish to add in some flexibility, so that it is permissible to break the rule if following it would lead to 'bad consequences'. A rule might be that all children should be vaccinated against measles to ensure that no one contracts measles or suffers from the complications of measles. However, some children do experience side effects from vaccination, so there may be grounds in some cases not to vaccinate an individual child, but ultimately policy decisions about this require a balance between outcomes for the individual and for the population as a whole. Thus, decisions are based on the consequences of not vaccinating or vaccinating. Therefore, once this qualification is added, it implies that the rule is not hard and fast and may be ignored – in particular, it can be ignored when the *consequences* are taken into account, and therefore rule utilitarianism appears to collapse back into act utilitarianism. The only way to preserve the difference between rule utilitarianism and act utilitarianism is to insist that the rules be obeyed *without exception*. In this case, even if following the rule will produce bad consequences, the rule utilitarian must follow them, regardless of the consequences – and therefore is no longer a consequentialist, and no longer a utilitarian.

When we come to apply utilitarianism to public health interventions, this becomes even more complicated. Common sense would seem to suggest that for any public health intervention to be considered ethical, the intervention must benefit the majority of 'all who are in any way affected' and harm as few as possible. On strict utilitarian grounds, this could be achieved through coercion, for example by passing legislation that forces people to adopt practices against their will (such as mandatory vaccination) or be tested or screened against their will (for example, genetic testing of infants) even in the face of (perhaps quite severe) harm to some. Furthermore, it is feasible that certain medical practices could be conducted on unwilling research 'guinea pigs' if it were believed to be in the interests of society (or at least of 'those who are in any way affected'). In public health policy, then, it would seem imperative to be able to calculate and define harm and benefit. How is this to be achieved? With utilitarianism we need to be able to quantify benefits in order to show that we have achieved the maximum well-being or good and that this outweighs any harm. The ethical and philosophical literature has amply explored these issues in relation to the moral right to restrict the actions and liberties of others in public health, based on discussion of utility, consequentionalism and rights (Mackie, 1977; Hare, 1982).

However, leaving these debates to one side, one key problem with public health policy and practice is the way in which benefit and harm are identified and measured. It seems obvious to say that public health policy and action should improve the overall well-being of the population. But this may, as in the case of vaccination, be to the detriment of some individuals' well-being. In order to justify vaccination programmes we therefore need to measure and compare, or balance out, these harms and benefits, even though it is not always clear that all benefits and harms are known about – or in other words, even though we may not have perfect information. As Cribb argues: "Given the complex causal and constitutive links between aspects of health, welfare, and well-being ... evaluations [of the effects of interventions], as well as the predictions they rest upon, have to be multidimensional" (Cribb, 2005, p 66). Essentially, there are four areas of balance that need to be addressed in public health:

- benefit and harm
- future benefit/harm over present benefit/harm
- individual or the population
- individual freedom or responsibility to protect the rights and freedoms of others.

These raise questions of definition and measurement. The role of an ethical framework is to guide decision making to provide the correct or best balance. The extent to which any one area is seen as more important than another will need to be reflected in the way judgements are made. The following section therefore explores the role of evidence in public health and discusses some of the methodological issues that arise in the way evidence is constituted and used in policy and practice.

Evidence-based public health policy and practice

Concern about the use of research and its influence on policy practice is not new (Weiss, 1979; Oliver, 2006). However, while it is increasingly being recognised that there are valid concerns about the basis and nature of evidence-based medicine, little attention has been paid to the area of public health policy.

Evidence is by nature contestable. In healthcare and medicine the dominant concept of evidence is that encapsulated in evidence-based medicine (EBM). This approach focuses on the individual patient and evidence is "developed through systematic and methodologically rigorous clinical research, emphasising the use of science and de-emphasising the use of intuition, unsystematic clinical experience, patient and professional values, and patho-psychologic rationale" (Dobrow et al, 2004, p 207). Critics of EBM argue that the approach is too narrow and excludes other forms of clinically relevant evidence (Miles et al, 2001). Proponents of EBM have responded by developing hierarchies of evidence based on methodological rigour, but these remain value bound and are not themselves evidence based (Ball et al, 2001; Miles et al, 2001). Despite these debates, EBM has continued to expand into clinical decision making and, increasingly, into the health policy arena, focusing attention on evidence-based health policy (Nutley and Davies, 2000; Black, 2001; Dobrow et al, 2004). Yet, as Black (2001) has argued "evidence-based policy is not simply an extension of EBM: it is qualitatively different".

Public health, by its very nature, is not focused on the individual but on populations, and the practice of public health is a more political process than medicine, as it deals with social processes and the wider population (Hunter, 2003). Values are more explicit in relation to public health than medical practice, although values are an important element of any system of healthcare. For example, the relative priority given to health inequalities is underpinned by ideological positions about the nature of inequality itself. Also, the debate about the extent to which the state should intervene in individual life-styles is not one that is open to a strictly evidence-based approach without recourse to some moral or ideological standpoint. However, evidence is often employed in arguments to sustain particular viewpoints (such as smoking, wearing seat belts, vaccination programmes).

Traditionally, public health has relied on epidemiological studies to demonstrate the need for and the effectiveness of interventions. These studies are designed to show that there has been an overall benefit from particular interventions. However, epidemiological evidence is not always clear, as demonstrated in recent debates about the effectiveness of the seasonal flu vaccination programmes. In some areas the evidence on effectiveness is much clearer (as in smallpox, polio), whereas in others questions are raised about who should be immunised (for example, influenza, TB). However, all immunisation programmes cause some harm to some individuals, but the effects to these individuals may not be statistically relevant in large-scale epidemiological studies, even though individual effects may be catastrophic. Therefore, leaving aside the broader politics for the present, decisions to introduce vaccination must be based on balancing the benefit to the many over harm to the few. However, the normal ways of identifying benefit and harm are not as clear cut as, say, testing a new drug, because the methodological issues of providing evidence are complex (Dobrow et al, 2004; Price et al, 2004). Dobrow et al (2004) suggest that evidence is either philosophical-normative (independent of context), with an emphasis on the quality and criteria for evidence, or practical-operational (context-based), where evidence "is characterised by its emergent and provisional nature, being inevitably incomplete and inconclusive" (p 209). The latter more accurately reflects the situation in public health, which relies on interpretation of evidence, such as in the debate about influenza deaths. Douglas (1986) has suggested, in fact, that in the way we make sense of the world, the categories of classification are all socially constituted and socially reproduced, and thus all evidence is set within specific contexts (or scientific paradigms: see Khun, 1969; Popper, 1970).

We can see how these perspectives relate to vaccination policy. Evidence about vaccine benefit and harm is collected through a variety of ways. However, initially vaccines are tested for effectiveness through clinical trials to demonstrate that they are safe and provide a specific outcome that confers benefit – usually identified as an observed immune response. The approach to clinical trials is rigorously monitored. Trials are, however, conducted on carefully screened patients who do not represent a 'normal' population. For example, vaccines are routinely tested on adults and dosages are adjusted by body mass for children. Also, it is thought that, as the immune systems of young children are not fully developed, higher dosages are required for very young children than might be given to an adult, in order to achieve an immune system response. There are also other unknowns, like the action and side effects of adjuvants. Evidence of effectiveness is also based on theoretical assumptions about how the immune system works, and there is no universal agreement on this (Matzinger, 2002). The actual safety of vaccines and population benefit rely on larger epidemiological studies and the collection of data on adverse events once the vaccine is in general use, but epidemiological studies may not be sensitive enough to identify problems, and reporting systems are not foolproof (Singleton et al 1999; Salisbury et al, 2002; Price et al, 2004). In cases where disease identification is clear (as in polio, TB) the population effect may be easy to identify, but in some areas, such as flu and flu-like symptoms, the situation is less clear, with considerable debate about the numbers of deaths from flu and the benefits of vaccination, based on interpretation of data extrapolated through assumptions about attributable deaths (Doshi, 2005; Jefferson, 2006). In all immunisation programmes there will also be individual instances of harm, and central to the identification of these are the adverse reaction reporting systems (the Yellow Card system in the UK), in which medical practitioners voluntarily report adverse effects of all drugs, including vaccines. However, the reliability of the system, while generally good, has suffered from under-reporting of adverse symptoms. It is thought that fewer than 10% are reported. Studies have shown that concerted attempts to make practitioners and patients aware of the need to report adverse events dramatically increase this figure.

As Davies (2005) and other authors demonstrate, there are a wide range of influences working on decision makers, of which formal research evidence is a small part (Oliver, 2006). One needs to recognise the context, competing interests and political processes that are involved in making policy. Research evidence is only one of a range of sources of evidence that are used by policy makers, and it competes with other sources of evidence. Public health policy making is being characterised by "bricolage" (Lévi-Strauss, 1966, pp 16–22), a process where the policy maker "in contrast to the scientist or engineer, acquires and assembles tools and materials as he or she goes, keeping them until they might be used" (Freeman, 2007). Moreover, as Lindblom and Cohen (1979) point out, evidence from research has to compete with "ordinary knowledge", which owes its origins to "common sense, casual empiricism or thoughtful speculation and analysis". In the specific case of health services, Hanney et al (2003) argue that there is generally more resistance to the use of social science than to the use of natural science, and they argue that natural science is less likely to incorporate political or ideological considerations. But this assumes that scientific evidence is not itself contestable, although it would be a brave politician indeed who suggested dismantling the vaccination programme – or the breast screening programme – on the grounds that it was based on 'bad' evidence, because there is a strong public perception that it is a public 'good'.

The ethical basis for vaccination

We are concerned in public health about the consequences of actions and the grounds upon which public health interventions can be justified. But little attention has been paid to how resultant harms and benefits are accounted for, and on what grounds public health interventions can be undertaken. This suggests some recourse to a set of rules or principles that do not bind actions, as in rule utilitarianism, or neglect how things are achieved, as in act utilitarianism.

However, before we go any further, we need to focus on the questions being asked here with regard to vaccination programmes. First, is it a 'good' policy; second, is it based on sound medical evidence; and third, is it 'good' for society?

With regard to the first question, whether or not something is a good policy depends, as Wildavsky (1972) has observed, on "who is doing the judging, what yardsticks they use, and on the basis of what information". Bearing this in mind, if public health policies are judged on the basis of their perceived benefits and whether or not they have public (and political) support, then vaccination is widely considered to be a 'good' policy. If we are to be cynical, what seems to be crucial in securing both public and political support in any public health policy is not just its substance, but how it looks (Hann, 1999a). Political judgements are more often than not based on impressions about the effects and costs of the programme, especially in the case of technical areas where specialised knowledge is needed in order to understand the complexities of possible costs and benefits. Coupled with this, policies become entrenched, and the political consequences of dismantling an ineffective programme that has strong public support may be greater than the consequences of leaving it in place. However, public support of health policies (such as vaccination or screening) is based on the belief that they (the public) are being correctly informed of the possible harms and benefits. However, as has been demonstrated elsewhere, the communication of risks and benefits is sometimes manipulated for political reasons (Skrabanek, 1994; Furedi, 1998; Hann, 1999b), and the medical evidence may not be as uncontroversial as people are led to believe.

This brings us to the second question: is the programme based on sound medical evidence? As was noted above, this issue is complicated. The drive for health promotion has brought with it a kind of obsession to vaccinate. Along with the already scheduled childhood vaccinations (diphtheria, polio, whooping cough, measles, rubella, tetanus, mumps, meningitis, pneumococcus, septicaemia and seasonal flu) there are suggestions that it might be advisable to routinely vaccinate against sexually transmitted infections, herpes, chickenpox and even bird flu. While the medical epidemiological evidence for some of these may be sound, for others it is less so and the focus on vaccination may even deflect attention from the broader social causes of infection (Herceg et al, 1994).

Third, whether or not a particular health policy is good for a particular society (as a whole) is a difficult and complex question, which turns on the precise definition of a 'good' (and 'society'), and the values that underpin it. All of which leaves us with a dilemma which, it seems, cannot be solved for us by utilitarianism (act or rule).

If the aim of public health policy is to reduce deaths and morbidity from disease x, the ends cannot justify the means if we want to live in a society that values individual autonomy, justice (however conceived) and informed choice. In addition, people can make genuine mistakes based on the best available information and with the best of intentions; policies come into being which are later found to be ineffective, inappropriate or counterproductive. If we are to abandon utilitarianism, how are we to judge the ethical merits of any given public health policy? One possibility is that proposed by Rosalind Hursthouse (and others) which invokes a notion of virtue. Her formulation of virtue ethics has its roots in the Aristotelian idea of 'moral character' or 'virtue'. While it is beyond the remit of this chapter to discuss virtue ethics in detail we can outline briefly how it might help us out of the quandary mentioned above. First, it is agent centred rather than act (or rule) centred. As Hursthouse puts it, virtue ethics addresses "itself to the question 'What sort of person should I be?' rather than to the question 'What sorts of action should I do?'" (p 17). So, while the utilitarian might claim that "an action is right if it promotes the best consequences", virtue ethics would instead claim that: "an action is right if it is what a virtuous agent would characteristically do in the circumstances".[5] While Hursthouse is reluctant to provide readers with a list of virtues, in the area of medical practice Beauchamp and Childress (1994) provide us with a possible starting point. They suggest that what Hursthouse calls virtues could just as easily be called 'principles', and these are: respectfulness, non-malevolence, benevolence, justice or fairness, truthfulness and confidentialness (p 67). Oakley and Cocking (2001) also list truthfulness, and add trustworthiness to the list of 'medical virtues' (p 93). However, this approach is not without its difficulties, and while many of the philosophical problems need not be discussed in detail here, one that we might mention is that these virtues may also be in tension or conflict with each other. General practitioners (for example) might have to put the patient's individual need above the needs of 'the many', for example by recommending that a particular child ought not to be vaccinated because of some pre-existing condition that is contra-indicated. As Hare (1993) points out: "Doctors in general tend to give extra weight to the interests of their own patients." Put into this context, might the actions of the virtuous general practitioner be in tension with the virtuous public health policy maker? However, leaving this aside for the moment, one way to apply virtue ethics in this instance is suggested by Oakley and Cocking (2001) in their book *Virtue ethics and professional roles*. They suggest that:

> One of the strengths of an approach to professional roles which takes their moral status to depend on importantly their links with key human goods is that this sort of approach fits naturally with a central feature of any occupations claim to be a profession in the first place. (p 79)

That is, we expect professionals – medical or political – to act in a 'professional' manner, which embraces a notion of acting morally within the context of their profession. We need to be able to rely on health professionals (and policy makers) to be *virtuous in their actions* in that they don't manipulate information, drown out opposing voices and ride roughshod over people's rights and autonomy.

Conclusion

An ethical approach to vaccination would, therefore, be one that demonstrated:

• that the intervention does what it says it is supposed to do
• that there is good medical evidence to support it

- that the harms and the benefits caused by the intervention are honestly and correctly understood and disseminated
- that alternative policy options are considered openly.

However, as the discussion earlier in the chapter highlights, there are questions that remain unanswered, including whether some vaccines 'do what they say they do'. An example here is the seasonal flu vaccine, where there is some debate about both efficacy and target populations (Jefferson, 2006). In addition, quantifying harm and benefit is difficult where evidence is contradictory or of a questionable standard (Price et al, 2004).

At the same time, vaccination is considered to be a social norm – it has wide social acceptability, strong political and medical support, and is widely seen as beneficial. Those questioning vaccination and vaccination policy are seen as 'cranks', anti-science, or simply ill-informed. Public support for vaccination programmes is paramount, given the need to reach a situation of herd immunity. This makes the furore over the MMR vaccination interesting. In order to ensure continued public support, a move to single vaccines might have been one way of keeping public confidence and high levels of immunisation rates. While supply of single vaccines was clearly an issue, this was a situation where a policy shift *not* based on evidence of improved efficacy might have been more useful rather than reliance on medical and scientific evidence showing that MMR was safe. In the case of the secondary school TB booster programme, strenuous efforts to ensure that all children were vaccinated – including pressure on parents who declined to have their children vaccinated – continued right up to the point of abandoning the programme on the basis of a review of evidence in 2005.

Vaccination programmes are undertaken within the context of competing values where evidence, individual freedom, practicality, political expediency, and support and different conceptualisation of harms and benefits coexist (Cribb, 2005; Salmon and Omer, 2006). There is also a degree of uncertainty about the nature of vaccination and the way in which it actually works. What is clear here is that a rational framework for deciding what course of action to take, based on best evidence, does not exist. Policy makers and practitioners are more often than not operating in an area of healthcare that does not conform to medical scientific paradigms. The adage that public health is politics is clearly pertinent, and developing an ethical framework for action must, necessarily, be set within a social context (Cribb, 2005).

Notes

[1] Immunisations give external benefits. When you receive a vaccine for a certain disease, it less likely that you will contract that disease (internal benefit), but it is also less likely that other people will contract the disease, because they will not catch it from you (external benefit). Most vaccines are not 100% effective, that is, they do not reduce the probability of contracting the disease, if one is exposed, to zero; but if a high percentage of the population receives the vaccine, a disease can be eradicated because those few people who have the disease may not happen to come into contact with an unvaccinated person.

[2] An individual in this case benefits from the immunisations that other people receive, because their actions reduce the risk of contacting someone with the disease. The free rider saves him/herself the risk of being immunised, but still reaps the benefits of the public health measure.

[3] This imperfect information can apply to both the individual and the policy maker. Controversies over medical evidence may be ignored, glossed over or even suppressed.

[4] Another common formulation of this premise is "the greatest happiness for the greatest number", but this is actually misleading. As Kymlicka observes, this contains two distinct maximands: 'greatest happiness' and 'greatest number'. It is impossible for any theory to contain a double maximand, and any attempt to implement it quickly leads to an impasse. See Griffin (1986, pp 151–4).

[5] Readers can find a more detailed discussion of virtue ethics in Foot (1978) and Hursthouse (1999).

References

Ball, C., Sackett, D., Philipps, B., Haynes, B., Straus, S. and Dawes, M. (2001) *Oxford Centre for Evidence-based Medicine Levels of Evidence*, (www.cebm.net/index.aspx?o=1025).

Beauchamp, T. and Childress, J. (1994) *Principles of biomedical ethics* (4th edn), Oxford: Oxford University Press.

Black, N. (2001) 'Evidence based policy: proceed with care', *British Medical Journal*, vol 323, pp 275–9.

Cribb, A. (2005) *Health and the good society*, Oxford: Oxford University Press.

Davies, P. (2005) 'Survey of senior Whitehall policy makers', presented by Dr Davies, Deputy Director, Chief Social Researcher's Office, Prime Minister's Strategy Unit, at a Workshop on 'Conducting and Commissioning Syntheses for Managers and Policy Makers', December, Montreal, Canada.

Dobrow, M., Goel, V. and Upshur, R. (2004) 'Evidence-based health policy: context and utilisation' *Social Science and Medicine*, vol 58, pp 207–17.

Doshi, P. (2005) 'Are flu death figures more PR than science?', *British Medical Journal*, vol 331, p 1412.

Douglas, M. (1986) *How institutions think*, Syracuse, NY: Syracuse University Press.

Foot, P. (1978) *Virtues and vices*, Berkeley, CA: University of California Press.

Freeman, R (2007) 'Epistemological bricolage: how practitioners make sense of learning', *Administration and Society*, vol 39, no 4, pp 476-96.

Furedi, F. (1998) *Culture of fear: Risk-taking and the morality of low expectation*, London: Cassell.

Griffin, J. (1986) *Well-being: Its meaning, measurement, and moral importance*, Oxford: Oxford University Press.

Guardian (2001) 'Court orders girls to have MMR jab', 13 June.

Hann, A. (1999a) 'Cancer test smeared: preventive medicine or an expensive mistake?', *Critical Public Health,* vol 9, no 3, pp 251–6.

Hann, A. (1999b) 'Propaganda versus evidence based health promotion: the case of breast screening', *International Journal of Health Planning and Management*, vol 14, pp 329-34.

Hanney, S., Gonzalez-Bloch, M., Buxton, M. and Kogan, M. (2003) 'The utilisation of health research in policy-making: concepts, examples and methods of assessement', *Health Research Policy and Systems*, vol 1, no 2. Available at www.health-policy-systems.com/content/1/1/2.

Hare, R.M. (1982) 'Ethical theory and utilitarianism', in A. Sen and B. Williams (eds) *Utilitarianism and beyond*, Cambridge: Cambridge University Press.

Hare, R. (1993) *Essays on bioethics*, Oxford: Oxford University Press.

Herceg, A., Pessaris, I. and Mead, C. (1994) 'An outbreak of measles in a highly immunised population: immunisation status and vaccine efficiency', *Australian Journal of Public Health*, vol 18, pp 249–52.

Hunter, D.J. (2003) *Public health policy*, Cambridge: Polity Press.

Hursthouse, R. (1999) *On virtue ethics*, Oxford: Oxford University Press.

Jansen,V., Stollenwerk, N., Jensen, H., Ramsay, M. et al (2003) 'Measles outbreaks in a population with declining vaccine uptake', *Science*, vol 301, p 804.

Jefferson, T. (2006) 'Influenza vaccination: policy versus evidence', *British Medical Journal*, vol 333, pp 912–15.

Kenny, N. and Giacomini, M. (2005) 'Wanted: A new ethics field for health policy analysis', *Health Care Analysis*, vol 13, no 4, pp 247–60.

Khun, T.S. (1969) 'Second thoughts on paradigms: Symposium on the structure of scientific theories', in F. Soppes (comp) (1977) *The structure of scientific theories*, Champaign, IL: University of Illinois Press.

Kymlicka, W. (1990) *Contemporary political philosophy: An introduction*, Oxford: Clarendon Press.

Lévi-Strauss, C. (1966) *The savage mind*, London: Weidenfeld and Nicholson.

Lindblom, C. and Cohen, D. (1979) *Usable knowledge: Social science and social problem solving*, New Haven, CT: Yale University Press.

Mackie, J.L. (1977) *Ethics: Inventing right and wrong*, London: Penguin.

Matzinger, P. (2002) 'The danger model: A renewed sense of self', *Science*, vol 296, pp 301–5.

Merck Sharp and Dohme (2006) Datasheet, M-M-R 11, measles mumps and rubella virus vaccine live, 015ml subcutaneous injection. DP/1-MMR-11–0206(280206).

Miles, A., Bentley, P., Polychronis, A., Grey, J., Melchiorri, C. (2001) 'Recent developments in the evidence-based healthcare debate', *Journal of Evaluation in Clinical Practice*, vol 7, no 2, pp 85–9.

Mill, J.S. (1974) *On liberty*, London: Penguin Classics.

Nutley, S. and Davies, H. (2000) 'Making a reality of evidence-based practice: some lessons from the diffusion of innovations'. *Public Money & Management*, vol 20, no 4, pp 35–42.

Oakley, J. and Cocking, D. (2001) *Virtue ethics and professional roles*, Cambridge: Cambridge University Press.

Oliver, T.R. (2006) 'The politics of public health policy', *American Review of Public Health*, vol 27, pp 195–233.

Popper, K. (1970) 'Normal science and its dangers', in I. Lakatos and A. Musgrave (eds), *Criticism and the growth of knowledge*, Cambridge: Cambridge University Press, pp 51–8.

Price, D., Jefferson, T. and Demicheli, V. (2004) 'Methodological issues arising from systematic reviews of the evidence of safety of vaccines', *Vaccine*, vol 22, pp 2080–4.

Salisbury, D.M., Beverley, P.C.L. and Miller, E. (2002) 'Vaccine programmes and policies', *British Medical Bulletin*, vol 62, pp 201–11.

Salmon, D.A. and Omer, S.B. (2006) 'Individual freedoms versus collective responsibility: immunization decision-making in the face of occasionally competing values', *Emerging Themes in Epidemiology*, vol 3, no 13. Available at www.ete-online.com/content/3/1/13.

Singleton, J.A., Lloyd, J.C., Mootrey, G.T. et al. (1999) 'An overview of the Vaccine Adverse Event Reporting System (VAERS) as a surveillance system', *Vaccine*, vol 7, pp 2908–17.

Skrabanek, P. (1994) *The death of humane medicine and the rise of coercive healthism*, London: Social Affairs Unit.

Weiss, C. (1979) 'The many meanings of research utilization', *Public Administration Review*, vol 39, pp 426–31.

WHO (World Health Organization) (2005) *Immunisation against diseases of public health importance: The benefits of immunisation*, factsheet no 288, Geneva: World Health Organization.

Wildavsky, A. (1972) 'The self-evaluating organization', *Public Administration Review*, vol 32, no 5, pp 509–20.

TEN

Avoiding mixed messages: HPV vaccines and the 'cure' for cervical cancer

Alison Hann and Stephen Peckham

Most vaccination programmes are concerned with reducing the prevalence and incidence of a particular infectious disease, such as TB or smallpox. The human papillomavirus (HPV) vaccine, however, is a vaccine that is designed to prevent the development of cervical cancer by protecting the individual against infection by HPV. This chapter examines the evidence base for the policy of a HPV vaccination programme, and suggests that the way in which this information is communicated to the public is loaded and that, furthermore, it may have serious consequences for the screening programme that could, arguably, be counterproductive.

Introduction

In the autumn of 2008 the UK government commenced the first wave of HPV vaccinations as part of a national programme aimed at 12- and 13-year-old girls. This is to be supplemented with a programme aimed at 18-year-old women. The instigation of the UK programme follows the lead of other countries – specifically the US and Canada – as part of a campaign to tackle cervical cancer. Since the announcement that the UK's Joint Committee on Vaccination and Immunisations recommended a vaccination programme, there has been extensive media coverage aimed at promoting the vaccine in the UK. While the programme is voluntary, it is being undertaken in secondary schools and there is substantial pressure on parents through media reports, celebrity endorsement and TV advertising to agree to the vaccination of their daughters. It is assumed that there is universal support for the vaccine and programme and it is being promoted as the cure for cervical cancer. However, such an approach mixes a number of key public health issues related to the purpose of the programme, who is being given protection, the interaction between different public health programmes and so on, that place public health practitioners and others involved in health promotion and public health in a difficult position.

While the HPV vaccine offers some hope of reducing the levels of cervical cancer, concerns have been expressed about its efficacy and the usefulness of the vaccination programme. This is an issue particularly with regard to long-term effects and side effects, and there is concern over the fact that it only protects against four out of the 200 HPV types. For this reason the vaccine does not confer 100% protection and there is still a need to have a national screening programme, particularly for older women. All cancer screening programmes almost inevitably result in a degree of unnecessary intervention (or in lack of intervention), due to the levels of sensitivity or specificity of tests, and this can be costly not only in terms of public spending but also in terms of personal anxiety and distress (Fahey et al, 1995; Dyer, 2003; Raffle et al, 2003).

In this chapter we consider some of the uncertainties associated with the 'control' of cervical cancer in the UK. In order to do this, we will consider both the current cervical cancer screening programme, and whether there may be good grounds for being cautious about a programme of vaccinations for HPV. We raise both questions about the efficacy of the programmes and ethical issues associated with screening and vaccine-based prevention programmes. We argue that these require serious consideration on the part of those responsible for public health programmes if clear public health messages are to be given to women, and in order to limit the potential negative impacts of the vaccination programme.

In 2004, 2,726 women in the UK were diagnosed with cervical cancer and in 2006, 949 women died (Cancer Research UK, 2007). This is despite a long-established cervical cancer screening programme – although rates are 70% lower than 30 years ago. The aetiology of cervical cancer is well understood and infection by HPV is recognised as being the most significant cause of cervical cancer as well as being associated with a number of less prevalent cancers (such as anal, vulvar, vaginal, penile head and neck cancers) and genital warts. It is not surprising, therefore, that the promise of an HPV vaccine led to widespread media coverage. On 1 June 2007, the *Guardian* newspaper ran a story entitled 'Cervical cancer vaccine for all women could cut cases by half', and it was not alone: most of the newspapers ran similar stories in the wake of the Department of Health's decision to accept (in principle) the recommendations of the Joint Committee on Vaccination and Immunisations (JCVI) that: "HPV vaccines should be introduced routinely for girls aged around 12–13 years" (JCVI, 2007). The decision was greeted with (almost) universal approval, and most reports quoted

Angela Raffle (of the UK Specialist Public Health Doctors' Group) as saying that the vaccine was a "fantastic breakthrough". Some reports were more enthusiastic than others – most reproduced the official figure that the vaccine protects against the HPV types that cause 70% of cervical cancers, while others made more extravagant claims. The *Sun*, for example, claimed that "the most feared cancers would be beaten within two generations". Enthusiasm over a vaccine that can protect against such a serious condition is perhaps to be expected. But is such enthusiasm really justified?

Cervical cancer screening

Enthusiasm for cervical cancer screening has grown almost unabated for almost 40 years, and it has been claimed that 100,000 lives have been saved since the programme began (Peto et al, 2004). The programme has had general cross-party political support and is now part of the primary care 'package' of health screening in the UK. In England the programme is estimated to cost approximately £157 million a year, and in Wales £7.9 million a year. In England four million women annually are routinely screened and for Wales the figure is 220,000. Cervical cancer screening is undertaken predominantly within general practice by GPs and practice nurses. In order to encourage practices to undertake the tests, practices have been offered financial incentives to achieve target rates of coverage. Between 1990 and 2004 practices were given financial incentives to achieve 50% and 80% coverage rates, and this did increase coverage, from 53% to 83% of GPs achieving the 80% target (Austoker, 1994; Langham et al, 1995). However, for GPs and practices which found it difficult to achieve even a 50% coverage, there was no real incentive to try to maximise the uptake of screening (Austoker, 1994). Since 2004, payments for cervical cancer screening have been made as part of the Quality Outcomes Framework (QOF) element of the new General Medical Services contract, which provides financial incentives to meet a range of clinical, organisational and patient experience criteria – worth approximately £125,000 per annum for a practice if maximum points are achieved. Early analysis of QOF has demonstrated that practices can achieve targets for activities rewarded through QOF to gain maximum income, although there are concerns about its negative impact on inequalities (McClean et al, 2006). In addition, questions have been raised concerning the ethics of incentivising GP practices to increase take-up rates for smear tests. For example, in order to encourage women to come forward for screening, the publicity programmes have been providing information that is in some cases misleading and in other cases just plain incorrect.

Current information concerning the cervical cancer screening programme may not be deliberate misinformation, but it certainly contains ambiguities. For example, the NHS Cervical Cancer Screening website clearly states that: "Cervical screening is *not* a test for cancer" (www.cancerscreening.nhs.uk/cervical/index.html, p 1). While the Forward to Shaping Futures *NHS Cervical Cancer Screening Service Report* (www.cancerscreening.nhs.uk.cervical/publications/cervical/annualreview) states: "Cervical screening is the only proven method of detecting cervical cancer" (p 3), other pamphlets describe the test as "detecting abnormal cells which are pre-cancerous", and the Cancer Research UK website states that the smear test "can detect cancer" (www.cancerresearch.org).

There is similar confusion over whether or not the cancer is sexually transmitted and over the risk of developing the disease if a woman has never been sexually active with a male partner. The Cervical Cancer Information Trust states clearly that cervical cancer is: "not transmitted via sexual intercourse" (p 13); while the Women's Health Forum has an information leaflet that states: "More than 90% of cervical cancers are transmitted through heterosexual sex"; and in another leaflet from the Women's Cancer Information Project, women are told that cervical cancer is caused by the HPV virus, which is passed on by an infected partner. Alongside this, women are being told that the disease is "extremely rare" in women under 25 (especially if they are not sexually active with a male), and yet are told they should attend for screening anyway. One of the consequences of the highly active campaign to recruit women into the programme has been the growing volume of litigation as a result of a false negative. In an editorial in the *British Medical Journal*, Wilson (2000) noted that:

> The enthusiasm of the health service to promote screening has perhaps given women unrealistic expectations. Women may falsely believe that screening prevents cancer. (p 1352)

The cervical cancer screening programme has had great success in promoting the benefits of the pap test, and while some efforts have recently been made by various organisations to be 'honest' with women concerning the possible drawbacks with screening, these tend to be rather downplayed, and the common perception is that cervical cancer is a disease that strikes almost indiscriminately at women of all ages and that it is a relatively common condition. Moreover, the risks associated with the test itself are also not so commonly understood by women who are encouraged to go for cervical screening tests. These are important considerations, and so we will briefly consider some of them here.

Cervical cancer is not a 'common condition'. Deaths from cervical cancer represent approximately 0.4% of all deaths in women, a fraction of the number of women who are diagnosed with or die from breast cancer. The JCVI report describes it as being "rare in England"; recent figures suggest that approximately 2,305 women a year will develop cervical cancer and, of these, about 950 will die because of it. While these deaths are tragic for the women concerned and their families, there is by no means an epidemic. Moreover, there are enormous variations in calculations of lives saved by the screening programme, varying between 800 and 4,500 lives saved every year (Raffle et al, 2003; Peto et al, 2004). The large variation in estimates of lives saved is a result of differing estimates of the incidence of HPV infection and calculations of future lives saved. While seemingly of a technical nature, such variations do have an important impact on determining both the effectiveness of the programme and its cost–effectiveness (Peto et al, 2004). The natural history of cervical neoplasia is not well understood, and although it has been estimated that about one third of cervical intraepithelial neoplasia (CIN) III will progress to invasive cancer if left alone, estimates of the time to progression and the rates of spontaneous regression for the various grades of CIN vary considerably. The test itself has never been assessed in a randomised controlled trial, and its introduction has been based primarily on observational studies. Furthermore, since the programme was implemented, women have been constantly urged to participate in it, and as a result the possibility of assessing the levels of costs and benefits through a randomised controlled trial have become ethically and practically impossible. While it certainly is true that both the incidence and mortality rates have been falling, the figures are difficult to interpret.

The test itself is not without difficulties. Estimates of the true sensitivity (true positive rate) range from 30% to 95%, but the most commonly quoted estimate of sensitivity is around 80% (Frame and Frame, 1998). Other difficulties with the test have been commented on by Wilson and Lister (2002), who point out that its sensitivity is strongly influenced by such things as procedures used during the collection and processing of samples, and increased sensitivity (reduction in the sampling and interpretation of samples) may be at the expense of decreased specificity by increasing the numbers of false positives. In addition, the calculation of sensitivity is further complicated because neither the number of true positives nor the number that would progress to invasive disease are known. The positive predictive value (PPV) of a screening test is often more clinically useful than sensitivity, because it shows the probability of a disease actually being present in those women with a positive test result. A single smear showing moderate dyskarosis or worse has a PPV for a diagnosis of CIN III or worse of 72%, while persistent inadequate, mild or borderline smears have a PPV of only 20% (DH, 2000). But over-diagnosis is not the only problem. One study found that the rate for false negatives for cervical cancer screening could be as high as 30% (Petticrew et al, 2001). The issue of sensitivity is a very important one, as the level of false positives has emotional and financial costs, and increasing levels of both false positives and false negatives have been the cause of litigation – something we will come back to later. A recent study by Raffle et al (2003) found that for every 10,000 women screened 10 deaths are probably avoided,[1] although these figures have been disputed by Peto and colleagues (Peto et al, 2004). However, Raffle et al (2003) argued that to prevent these 10 deaths 1,564 women are referred for "further investigations" which could include anything from a simple repeat smear to colposcopy or biopsy. The study noted that cervical cancer screening involves treatment for many women who are not destined to develop invasive cancer and that there is a risk of iatrogenic harm. Furthermore, another study carried out by Fahey et al (1995) observed that new technologies have the potential to increase costs even further by increasing the identification of even more minor abnormalities.

While it is clear that the cervical screening programme has saved the lives of many women the programme is far from perfect. However, as it has been running for nearly 40 years and has wide political, professional and public support, substantive changes to the programme or questioning of its effectiveness are likely to be very limited. In addition there appears to be some confusion about issues of risk, the impact of the programme and how incentives for screening impact on how the programme operates. A key question must be, however, whether the recent proposals for tackling HPV provide substantial improvements to the screening programme.

Human papillomavirus vaccines

Cervical cancer is the first cancer shown to be caused by an infection, which is preventable by a vaccine. However, although HPV infection is necessary for cervical cancer to develop and the vaccine may prevent primary infection with HPV types 16 and 18 (associated with most cervical cancer cases – in the US it is 50.5% and 13.1% respectively), it has been estimated that jointly HPV 16 and 18 account for 70% of cervical cancers (Munoz et al, 2003; Dunne et al, 2007) and this figure is the most widely quoted, although there are geographical and population variations in rates of HPV infection (Wright et al, 2006). There are nearly 200 types of HPV, of which 15 are associated with cervical cancer (Zimmerman, 2006). However, the epidemiology of HPV is not straightforward. It is true that exposure within a few years of commencing sexual activity is common. The incidence of HPV among young women in the US has been thought to be as high as 54% (Winer et al, 2003); the incidence for types 16 and 18 is significantly lower – between 7% and 10.4%, and 4% and 4.1%, respectively (Ho et al, 1998; Winer et al, 2003), and Dunne et al (2007) in their US study of women aged 14 to 59 concluded that while "the burden of prevalent HPV infection among women was higher than previous estimates … the prevalence of HPV vaccine types was relatively low" (p 819). In addition, rates vary by age, and most HPV infections are asymptomatic and only persistent infection over a long period leads to cervical cancer (Zimmerman, 2006).

The new vaccine by Merck Inc. (Gardasil), has been shown to be highly effective against HPV 16 and 18, and that by GlaxoSmithKline to be similarly effective (Harper et al, 2004; Villa et al, 2005). However, as Laurance (2007) points out, while some have claimed that the vaccine has a 99% success rate, this is highly misleading: "A 99 per cent 'success rate' against the two commonest causes does not mean a 99 per cent protection against cervical cancer. It means, according to the trial results, about a 70% protection. Thus any girl who had the vaccination would, once she became sexually active, still have a 30 per cent chance of being infected with another HPV virus which could develop into cancer." However, while infection with HPV is necessary for the development of cervical cancer, infection does not lead inevitably to cancer. Indeed, as stated above, most HPV infections clear spontaneously. Recent research has suggested that clearance occurs within one year for about 70% of infected women, and within two years for 90% (Public Health Agency of Canada, 2007). It is therefore important not to conflate HPV and cervical cancer. This is something that is recognised in the JCVI (2007) report: "so the actual incidence of HPV cannot be accurately determined…. it also takes about 6–12 months for an incident of HPV infection to produce an antibody response … and there are studies which show that in women with cervical cancer, only 50% are seropositive (p 6).

Another important question needs to be raised about a population-based HPV vaccination programme, and that concerns the exact target that the Department of Health has in mind. Is it to eradicate the high-risk types of HPV from the population? Or is the aim to reduce the number of deaths from cervical cancer? This is important, because these two goals require different strategies and impact on cost-effectiveness (Ferko et al, 2008). If the goal is the elimination of HPV types 16 and 18, then this requires herd immunity, and this would require the vaccination of boys, because while boys (males) do not suffer from cervical cancer they do carry the virus that causes it. Interestingly, in the same report mentioned above, herd immunity is only referred to once, and that is with regard to genital warts, which are also caused by HPV in both men and women. It states: "the additional benefits in vaccinating boys to reduce the incidence of warts is low. This is because with a sustained high vaccine coverage in women, eventually all cases of warts would be eliminated because of herd immunity and the indirect protection of men"(p 7). This is an important consideration, as the calculation of the cost-effectiveness of the vaccination programme is based on calculations of not just the prevention of cervical cancer, but also the cost to the NHS of treating genital warts in both males and females, although this is rarely mentioned in the newspaper articles. If, however, the aim of the vaccination programme is to reduce the number of deaths from cervical cancer, then it would seem to require a vaccine that targeted more than just two of the high-risk HPV types which are covered by Gardasil.

But there are other unanswered questions with regard to the usefulness of this vaccine. One is the length of the immunologic protection that it confers. The figure being used by the JCVI is 5 years, but this suggests that a booster may be necessary – otherwise girls who were vaccinated at 12 or 13 might reach their late teens (statistically, a period of high sexual activity) thinking that they are protected, when in fact they are not. There are also concerns about the short-term immunity altering the natural history of the viral infection, as seems to be the case with chickenpox (Chaves et al, 2007). If all this were not enough, there are still further difficulties. For example, there is not very much data concerning the effectiveness of the HPV vaccine when it is administered with other immunisations, and a number of questions have been raised concerning the methodologies and research findings of Merck, the company that makes Gardasil. These criticisms come from a variety of sources. One is taken up by Lippman et al (2007), who point out that "relatively few girls (about 1,200 aged 9–12 years) were enrolled in the clinical trials of Gardasil, the youngest of whom were only followed up for eighteen months.... Clearly this is thin information on which to construct a policy of mass vaccination" (p 177). Other methodological questions have been raised by Allen (2007) concerning Merck's policy of outsourcing clinical trials. Jayalan Pharmaceutical Research in India was one of the companies with which Merck had a contract to test Gardasil. Like many companies in the pharmaceutical industry, Merck increasingly outsources its clinical trials to contract research organisations (CROs) in areas of the world where trial subjects are plentiful, operating costs are low and regulations not so strict. The CROs are renowned for completing clinical trials in record times. Allen points out that "Conflicts of interest can arise when CROs are paid royalties only after a drug is approved rather than being paid a set fee that is independent of how safe or effective a drug turns out to be" (Allen, 2007). In addition to this, the National Vaccine Information Centre (NVIC) has stated that in its opinion "Merck and the FDA have not been completely honest with people about the pre-licensure clinical trials". The issue it is raising concerns the use of a potentially reactive aluminium-containing placebo as a control for most trial participants, rather than a non-reactive saline solution. They point out that a reactive placebo can artificially increase the appearance of safety of an experimental drug or vaccine in a clinical trial:

> Gardasil contains 225mcg of aluminium and although aluminium adjuvants have been used in vaccines for decades, they were never tested for safety in clinical trials. Furthermore, it seems that there has been a significant number of adverse reactions to both Gardasil and the placebo which have been 'dismissed' as 'unrelated' – these include 17 deaths and adverse events such as pain and swelling at the injection site and systemic effects such as headache, nausea, dizziness, gastroenteritis, asthma, juvenile arthritis and lupus (Fisher, 2006).

Another and perhaps more cynical line of criticism concerns the marketing methods used by Merck to promote its vaccine – both in the UK and the US. In US, questions have been raised concerning the social marketing of Gardasil directly to the public, while other commentators such as Allen (2007) have remarked upon the influence of groups such as Women in Government (WIG), a supposedly non-profit organisation which promotes 'women's issues' and which has been receiving sponsorship from Merck. The group has been heavily involved in lobbying on behalf of Merck to introduce bills in some 20 states to have vaccination with Gardasil made mandatory for girls aged as young as 9 years. Allen also points out that in the US Gardasil was fast-tracked for approval, that the FDA (US Food and Drug Administration) can fast-track drugs, but there is a charge. The FDA charges anywhere from $50,000 to nearly $900,000 to fast-track a drug; since 1992, drug companies have paid the FDA $1.7 billion to speed up the approval process for various drugs. This fast-tracking was perhaps especially important in this case, as a rival company, GlaxoSmithKline (GSK), was developing a similar vaccine. In the US, if Gardasil becomes routine (mandatory), it will generate annual sales of $3.2 billion by 2010 (Allen, 2007). In the UK the vaccine costs around £300 for the series of three doses and it was estimated that a full vaccination programme would cost the NHS roughly £120 million a year (Laurance, 2007). This makes it a very expensive vaccination. Actual vaccine costs are in fact lower, but rather than use the quadvalent Gardasil, the UK government has opted for the GSK bivalent Cervarix, which will cost only £8.9 million per year for the current vaccination programme – a saving of up to £18.6 million on the vaccine price alone. Interestingly, Cervarix was also hastened through the approval process, because of the pressure to compete with Gardasil. Such a decision implies that the government considers this saving worth more than any benefits of averting cases of genital warts (Kim, 2008). This is still expensive by vaccine standards, as, for example, the MMR vaccination costs £12 for the two doses. (It is worth noting here that private clinics in the UK are already advertising the availability of a course of injections – for example the Centre for the Prevention of HPV and Treatment of HPV Related Diseases in London is offering a course of three injections for £450). But the 'money trail' doesn't end there – Merck is still recovering from the Vioxx disaster. Vioxx was withdrawn last year after it was claimed to have caused the deaths of almost 28,000 people (Allen, 2007). None of this, of course, necessarily means that Gardasil is unsafe, and it is perfectly possible that Gardasil is everything that Merck claims that it is, but all the same it would be naive not to consider the wider forces at work, and the possible conflicts of interest.

But there is another issue that we have not yet tackled, and that is the relationship between the cervical cancer screening programme in the UK and the proposed vaccination programme for HPV. Angela Raffle has already expressed concerns that the vaccination programme may lead to women feeling that they are 'protected' and that this may cause the collapse of the screening programme. She comments that "for older women, the vaccine comes too late" and that they would still need to be screened (Curtis, 2007). But even for those girls who are vaccinated before exposure to HPV, this does not rule out infection from another one of the high-risk viruses, and these women would still need to be screened. This point is highlighted by the fact that the day after the UK government announced the start of the HPV vaccination programme the head of the cervical cancer screening programme appeared on national radio to urge women not to stop attending for cervical smears.

With the launch of the programme, some of these concerns about the programme and the vaccine are being identified in practice. In a study of coverage rates in a Manchester school, Brabin et al (2008) found that 70.6% of the girls received the first dose and 68.5% the second (no data is available on the third dose). This is lower than other school-based programmes (Waller and Wardle, 2008). The main concerns of the parents of those not receiving the vaccine were safety and efficacy. In the US and Canada major concerns have been raised about vaccinating young girls before they are sexually active – seen as condoning sexual activity – but this was not a concern that was raised in Brabin et al's study. One area that also needs further investigation is the question of competency of the girls themselves, and whether parental consent is required or whether girls of 12 and 13 are 'Gillick competent', raising important ethical issues for the girls, their families, the schools where school-based programmes are being used and the NHS (Brown, 2008; Waller and Wardle, 2008).

Conclusion

Where does this leave the campaign to combat cervical cancer? While the difficulties surrounding the pap smear test are not resolved, the difficulties that seem to be associated with the HPV vaccination programme would seem to suggest that it would be, at the very least, imprudent to abandon it. While there may still be issues concerning ways in which the negative (or possible iatrogenic) difficulties associated with the pap test are dealt with, the ways in which women are informed and recruited into the cervical cancer screening programme, and the related problems around possibly targeting those at a higher risk of developing the disease, there is also the worrying conundrum that the women most likely to suffer from cervical cancer are the ones who never attend for screening. Key risk indicators for persistent HPV infection and cervical cancer are, not surprisingly, similar. While HPV vaccination will undoubtedly lead to reductions in HPV infection, this is only true if full courses of vaccine are administered (currently a three-dose regime) and long-term efficacy is assured. Full protection will only be available to those who complete courses and return for boosters. Clearly, testing for HPV – especially types 16, 18, 52 and 58 – may provide a good test for predicting risk of cervical cancer (Ho et al, 2006). It is likely that the introduction of the new molecular approaches (based on enzyme or methylation testing) may be the answer here (Gravitt et al, 2008). The programme of HPV vaccination will lead to changes in cervical cancer screening, as the existing smear test is expensive and produces many incorrect results and the over-management of low-grade lesions.

Vaccination programme effectiveness would also need to be based on known rates of HPV infection, as cervical cancer can also be caused by strains other than those for which the vaccine provides protection. Studies in the US suggest that the incidence for types 16 and 18 is significantly lower than was previously thought, that infection rates vary by age and that most HPV infections are asymptomatic (Dunne et al, 1998; Winer et al, 2003; Ho et al, 2006; Zimmerman, 2006).

This is an important point when considering the primary prevention of cervical cancer and HPV infection. Cervical cancer is a sexually transmitted disease; as many as two-thirds of women who are infected with HPV will not develop cervical cancer. Primary prevention strategies that provide factual information regarding transmission of sexually transmitted infection (STI) and the teaching of safer sex negotiation skills are potentially highly effective, at a relatively low cost (Shepherd et al, 2000). Condom use has been shown to help prevent the transmission both of HPV and of other STIs (Winer et al, 2003).

Key questions arise, therefore, about whether universal vaccination is appropriate. The vaccine offers individual protection only if administered before sexual activity commences or where individuals are HPV free. Already in North America, where some US states and Canadian provinces are introducing programmes, concerns have been raised by conservative and religious groups about routine and mandatory vaccination, as they feel that this will lead to increased sexual activity (Zimmerman, 2006). While this may be an issue in the UK, the other main concerns mentioned above should be subject to further debate. Certainly the claims in the media about the efficacy of the vaccine and the potential eradication of cervical cancer bear little relation to the reality of what can be achieved with the current vaccination. However, on the current evidence, we would think twice before encouraging our daughters to be vaccinated.

More importantly, while of obvious benefit and importance, cervical cancer screening programmes and HPV vaccination are not in themselves totally effective strategies. Screening may detect early (or more advanced) lesions, but this is not without problems. Likewise, a population vaccination programme for HPV also raises questions that have, so far, not been answered satisfactorily. Primary prevention through education and promotion of safe sexual practices must, therefore, play a central role in any programme aimed at reducing cervical cancer deaths in the long term, but this appears to be sadly lacking within the UK's approach to cervical cancer. The challenge for public health practitioners and policy makers is to ensure that accurate messages about safety, transmission, efficacy and prevention are given to the public. This will involve a complex discussion with a range of key parties, including local community health services, schools, teachers, parents and the girls themselves.

Note
[1] Another way of expressing this is that screening 1,000 women for 35 years prevents one cervical cancer.

References
Allen, T. (2007) 'Merck's murky dealings: HPV vaccine lobby backfires', *Spinwatch*. Available at www.spinwatch.org/content/view/4080/9/ (accessed 9 August 2007).

Austoker, J. (1994) 'Screening for cervical cancer', *British Medical Journal*, vol 309, pp 241–7.

Brabin, L., Roberts, S.A., Baxter, D., Chambers, G., Kitchener, H. and McCann, R. (2008) 'Uptake of first two doses of human papillomavirus vaccine by adolescent schoolgirls in Manchester: prospective cohort study', *British Medical Journal*, vol 336, pp 1056–8.

Brown, E.C.F. (2008) 'Some issues around consent remain unresolved', *British Medical Journal*, vol 336, p 1146.

Cancer Research UK (2007) UK Cervical Cancer statistics website, http://info.cancerresearchuk.org/cancerstats/types/cervix/?a=5441 (accessed 24 August 2007).

Chaves, S.S., Gargiullo, P., Zhang, J.X., Civen, R., Guris, D., Mascola, L. and Seward, J.F. (2007) 'Loss of vaccine induced immunity to varicella over time', *New England Journal of Medicine*, vol 356, pp 1121–9.

Curtis, P. (2007) 'Cervical cancer vaccine for all women could cut cases by half – study', *Guardian*, 1 June.

DH (Department of Health) (2000) *Cervical Screening Programme, England: 1999–2002*, Department of Health Statistical Bulletin 2000/30, London: DH.

Dunne, E.F., Unger, E.R., Sternberg, M., McQuillan, G., Swan, D.C., Patel, S.S. and Markowitz, L.E. (2007) 'Prevalence of HPV infection among females in the United States', *Journal of the American Medical Association*, vol 297, no 8, pp 813–19.

Dyer, O. (2003) 'Government fails to meet targets for sexually transmitted infections', *British Medical Journal*, vol 326 (7395), p 900.

Fahey, M., Irwing, L. and Macaskill, P. (1995) 'Meta analysis of pap test accuracy', *American Journal Epidemiology*, vol 336, p 1180.

Ferko, N., Postma, M., Gallivan, S., Kruzikas, D. and Drummond, M. (2008) 'Evolution of the health economics of cervical cancer vaccination', *Vaccination*, vol 26S, pp F3–F15.

Fisher, B. (2006) 'Merck's Gardasil vaccine not proven safe for little girls'. Available at www.redorbit.com.

Frame, P.S. and Frame, J.S. (1998) 'Determinants of cancer screening frequency: the example of screening for cervical cancer', *Journal of the American Family Practitioner*, vol 11, pp 87–95.

Gravitt, P.E., Coutlee, F., Iftner, T., Sellors, J.W., Quint, W.G.V. and Wheeler, C.M. (2008) 'New technologies in cervical cancer screening', *Vaccine*, vol 265, pp K42–K52.

Harper, D., Franco, E., Wheeler, C. et al (2004) 'Efficacy of a bivalent L1 virus-like particle vaccine in prevention of infection with human papillomavirus types 16 and 18 in young women: a randomised controlled trial', *The Lancet*, vol 364, no 9447, pp 1757–65.

Ho, G.Y.F., Bierman, R., Beardsley, L., Chang, C.J. and Burk, R.D. (1998) 'Natural history of cervical human papillomavirus infection in young women', *New England Journal of Medicine*, vol 338, no 7, pp 423–8.

Ho, C.M., Chien, T.Y., Huang, S.H., Lee, B.H. and Chang, S.F. (2006) 'Integrated human papillomavirus types 52 and 58 are infrequently found in cervical cancer, and high viral loads predict risk of cervical cancer', *Gynecologic Oncology*, vol 102, no 1, pp 54–60.

JCVI (2007) 'Minutes of the HPV sub-group meeting, Wednesday 28 February 2007'. Available at www.advisorybodies.doh.gov.uk/jcvi/mins-hpv-280207.htm (accessed 9 August 2007).

Kim, J.J. (2008) 'Human papillomavirus vaccination in the UK', *British Medical Journal*, vol 337, pp 303–4.

Langham, S., Gillam, S. and Thorogood M. (1995) 'The carrot, the stick and the general practitioner: how have changes in financial incentives affected health promotion activity in general practice?', *British Journal of General Practice*, vol 45, pp 665–8.

Laurance, J. (2007) 'Is the new cervical cancer vaccine as good as it's claimed?', *Independent*, 12 June.

Lippman, A., Melnychuk, R., Shimmin, C. and Boscoe, M. (2007) 'Human papillomavirus, vaccines and women's health: questions and cautions', *Journal of the Canadian Medical Association*, 28 August, Available online at www.cmaj.ca.

McClean, G., Sutton, M. and Guthrie B. (2006) 'Deprivation and quality of primary care services: evidence for persistence of the inverse care law from the UK Quality and Outcomes Framework', *Journal of Epidemiology and Community Health*, vol 60, no 11, pp 917–22.

Munoz, N., Bosch, F.X., de Sanjosé S. et al (2003) 'Epidemiologic classification of human papillomavirus types associated with cervical cancer', *New England Journal of Medicine*, no 348, pp 518–27.

Peto, J., Gilham, C., Fletcher, O., and Mathews, F. (2004) 'The cervical cancer epidemic that screening has prevented in the UK', *The Lancet*, vol 364, no 9430, pp 249-56.

Petticrew, M., Sowden, A. and Lister-Sharp, D. (2001) 'False negative results in screening programmes: medical, psychological and other implications', *International Journal of Technology Assessment in Health Care*, vol 17, no 2, pp 164–70.

Public Health Agency of Canada (2007) 'What everyone should know about human papillomavirus (HPV): questions and answers'. Available at www.phac-aspc.gc.ca/std-mts/hpv-vph/hpv-vph-qaqr_e.html (accessed 19 July 2007).

Raffle, A., Alden, B., Quinn, M., Babb, P.J. and Brett, M.T. (2003) 'Outcomes of screening to prevent cancer: analysis of cumulative incidence of cervical abnormaility and modelling of cases and deaths prevented', *British Medical Journal*, vol 326, p 901.

Shepherd, J., Peersman, G., Weston, R. and Napuli, I. (2000) 'Cervical cancer and sexual lifestyle: a systematic review of health education interventions targeted at women', *Health Education Research*, vol 15, no 6, pp 681–94.

Villa, L.L., Costa, R.L.R., Petta, C.A. et al (2005) 'Prophylactic quadrivalent human papillomavirus (types 6, 11, 16 and 18) L1 virus-like particle vaccine in young women: a randomised double-blind placebo-controlled multi-centre phase II efficacy trial', *The Lancet*, vol 6, pp 271–8.

Waller, J. and Wardle, J. (2008) 'HPV vaccination in the UK', *British Medical Journal*, vol 336, pp 1028–9.

Wilson, R. (2000) 'Screening for breast and cervical cancer as a common cause for litigation', *British Medical Journal*, vol 320, pp 1352–3.

Wilson, S. and Lister, H. (2002) 'How can we develop a cost effective quality cervical cancer screening programme?', *British Journal of General Practice*, June, pp 485–90.

Winer, R.L., Lee, S.K., Hughes, J.P., Adam, D.E., Kiviat, N.B. and Koutsky, L.A. (2003) 'The epidemiology of human papillomavirus infections', *American Journal of Epidemiology*, vol 348, pp 518–27.

Wright, T.C., Bosch, F.X., Franco, E.L., Cuzick, J., Schiller, J.T., Garnett, G.P. and Meheus, A. (2006) 'Chapter 30: HPV vaccines and screening in the prevention of cervical cancer; conclusions from a 2006 workshop of international experts', *Vaccine*, vol 24S3, pp 251–61.

Zimmerman, R. (2006) 'Ethical analysis of HPV vaccine policy options', *Vaccine*, vol 24, pp 4812–20.

ELEVEN

A call for clearer vaccine exemption typology to improve population health

Erica Sutton and Ross Upshur

This chapter explores a central theme in public health ethics, namely, how far it is ethically defensible to use different forms of 'social influence' to ensure that individuals comply with immunisation policies that are designed to serve the good of the population. This rests on two main concerns: first, some kind of assessment of the health benefits of vaccination, and second, a consideration of the balance of individual autonomy and the good of the population.

Introduction

Eradicating communicable diseases has been a primary public health goal for centuries, and vaccination programmes comprise a significant part of that population health effort. To achieve community health, public health authorities are bestowed with policing powers whereby individual rights may be sacrificed for the greater good of the population (Mann et al, 1999; Gostin, 2004). However, healthcare providers and scholars are encouraging public health programmes to attain their community health goals through the least coercive and intrusive means possible (Gostin, 2004). The coercive strategies implemented by public health authorities in the past are discouraged today (Mann et al, 1999). Public health strategies that aim to balance individual and community rights and recognise that protecting human rights positively affects individual and population health are preferred (Mann et al, 1999). Despite a history of coercive strategies adopted by public health vaccination programmes, particularly in the US, vaccines have been deemed among the most successful public health interventions (Salmon and Siegel, 2001). However their success has been accompanied by controversy. Anti-vaccination movements have challenged state infringement of bodily integrity and individual rights since the nineteenth century and have been particularly vocal in countries mandating vaccination (Arnup, 1992; Colgrove, 2005; Blume, 2006; Salmon et al, 2006).

As population health threats emerge and as new vaccines are developed to address them, the ethical implications of vaccination programmes (particularly of mandatory vaccines) will be of increasing concern to individuals of all ages, cultures and ethnicities. As public health departments prepare their vaccination programmes for the future, an approach that recognises the importance of protecting individual human rights, as delineated in both the Universal Declaration of Human Rights (UDHR) (United Nations, 1948) and the 'Siracusa Principles' (ECOSOC, 1984), is a necessary first step towards ensuring the health of the community.

This chapter has four main objectives: the first is to offer concrete distinctions between the terminology used in immunisation discussions, such as 'compulsory', 'mandatory', 'religious', 'philosophical', 'personal' and 'conscientious'. The second is to demonstrate how the use of vaccination language serves to de-emphasise the role that public health departments have in individual decisions to object. The third aim is to explore whether and how the sincerity of conscientious objections can be proved, and the fourth to outline the public health advantages of adopting immunisation programmes that promote and protect human rights.

Mandatory vaccination versus voluntary vaccination

'Compulsory' and 'mandatory' are two terms used seemingly interchangeably to describe past and present vaccination programmes adopted in the US and elsewhere around the globe. Both adjectives convey a sense of obligation that suggests that opting out from immunisation is not available. In the late nineteenth century, opting out resulted in significant consequences: failing to subject oneself or one's child to compulsory vaccination resulted in a financial penalty, incarceration, quarantine or barring of entry into school (Colgrove, 2005; Gostin, 2005; Mariner et al, 2005). Although 'compulsory' and 'mandatory' are still used to characterise vaccination programmes, immunisation policies and practices have shifted over time.

Today, individuals are permitted to opt out for medical, religious or philosophical reasons without heavy penalties, provided that they complete an exemption form: such documentation may or may not require interaction with a healthcare provider or religious leader to confirm and validate the objection rationale (Salmon and Siegel, 2001; Wynia, 2007a). Wynia (2007a) maintains that labour-intensive exemption processes reflect the modern-day 'mandate': bureaucratic hoops are purposefully constructed to render opting out of vaccination more difficult and thus less appealing (p 3). Use of the term 'mandatory' is also a rhetorical strategy wielded in public health debates (Wynia, 2007a). Opponents of a given public health measure may label an intervention mandatory in order to incite ire in individuals who endorse libertarian philosophies (Wynia, 2007a). Critics also tend to label interventions that adopt opt-out, rather than opt-in, as mandatory policies (Wynia, 2007a). Conversely, proponents of a given public health intervention may invoke the term 'mandatory' to convey a sense of urgency and/or seriousness to the intervention, in order to elicit the desired uptake response by the public and insurers (Wynia, 2007a). However, rendering 21st-century vaccination programmes compulsory or mandatory may result in counteracting public health efforts, regardless of the perceived health effects attributed to the past successes of mandatory vaccination programmes. Specifically, the language and laws of compulsion publicly delineate the extent to which the state can infiltrate the most personal of private spheres: bodily integrity and child rearing (Colgrove, 2005). In the past, opposition to such invasions of privacy spawned the anti-vaccination movement, whose persistence ultimately contributed to the legal recognition of conscientious objections (Arnup, 1992).

Anti-vaccinationists typically exert their pressure where vaccination programmes are compulsory (Arnup, 1992; Colgrove, 2005; Salmon et al, 2006) and convey their messages through pamphlets, brochures and, more recently, the Internet (Zimmerman, 2004). Compulsion is one of the numerous reasons why individuals seek exemption from vaccination. Such opposition is based on principled objections against the role of the state, independent from the vaccine itself (Blume, 2006).

A public health strategy that implements compulsory immunisation programmes in the knowledge not only that individuals will object on principle and are legally protected to do so (Salmon et al, 2005) but also that anti-vaccination movements will resurface does little to achieve vaccination uptake goals. Moreover, given the emphasis placed on informed decision making in healthcare, vaccination programmes involving competent adults should be voluntary:

> Participation in vaccination programmes should, generally, be voluntary because of the importance now given to autonomous decision making by competent adults in health care. (Verweij and Dawson, 2004, p 3125)

The US Supreme Court has given public health officials significant leeway to preserve and protect community health at any cost (Gostin, 2005). However, human rights activists and scholars appeal to ethical norms and encourage public health authorities to use the least coercive means whenever possible to achieve health goals (Mann et al, 1999; Gostin, 2004; Mariner et al, 2005). For instance, if high levels of immunisation can be achieved through voluntary programmes, such programmes should be supported and implemented (Verweij and Dawson, 2004). Numerous countries boast successful voluntary programmes with high levels of immunity; among them are Sweden, Denmark, Norway, the Netherlands and the UK (Salmon et al, 2006). Such countries are significantly smaller in size and population than the US, and models that work in one country may not necessarily work in another. However, overall public support for vaccination in the US is strong and relatively few individuals refuse vaccines (Salmon and Siegel, 2001; Verweij and Dawson, 2004; Zimmerman, 2004). In addition, Salmon et al (2006) maintain that a successful mandatory immunisation programme requires mass public support: "For compulsory vaccination to work as planned, the great majority of the population must be willing to be vaccinated" (p 440). This raises the question whether, if a majority is needed to support a compulsory programme, that same majority would support a voluntary programme.

Exemption typology

Although most lay people allegedly support vaccination programmes (Zimmerman, 2004), exemptions are sought for various medical and non-medical reasons. Understanding the motivations behind such objections is critical for public health programme evaluation, offering an opportunity to identify public (mis)conceptions pertaining to immunisation and to explore ways of educating more effectively in the future. Further investigation into why individuals and parents refuse vaccinations is needed (Salmon and Siegel, 2001). However, some data do exist, and exemption rationales have been categorised and labelled as being either 'medical', 'religious', 'philosophical', 'personal' or 'conscientious'. An additional exemption category is introduced here that explicitly incorporates appeals based on barriers to access, labelled a 'structural barriers exemption'.

Aside from this addition, medical, religious, philosophical, personal and conscientious rationales are categories frequently used in the vaccination literature and often left undefined by scholars, who seem to assume a shared starting point. Consequently, philosophical, personal and conscientious motivations for exemption are often conflated and the terms used interchangeably, despite distinct differences evident in the scholarship. Adopting all-encompassing vaccine jargon to characterise exemptions can be perceived as a strategic effort to place the consequences of low vaccine uptake and the correlating increase in disease outbreaks with the 'quirky', 'irresponsible' or 'lazy' individual rather than considering objections to vaccination as indicative of a more systemic weakness in public health intervention programmes themselves.

Prior to outlining and challenging the various characteristics that comprise vaccination exemptions, this chapter proposes that 'conscientious objection' be the umbrella term under which specific non-medical exemptions fall – namely, religious, philosophical, personal and conscience-based exemptions. Social barrier exemptions would not fall under this broad category, given that exemptions based on limited financial resources and work constraints do not (at least on the surface) reflect an ethical or moral framework grounding the decision; these exemptions are made of necessity.

In addition, adopting consistent use of the term 'conscientious objector' would also mirror more closely the ongoing debate of the role of conscientious objection in medicine as discussed concerning healthcare providers. In that context, the phrase is interpreted as a difficult to define, conscience-based appeal that spans diverse religious, cultural and philosophical traditions (see Card, 2007; Lawrence and Curlin, 2007). Invoking the UDHR (United Nations, 1948) as a necessary part of public health offers additional support for conscience-based exemptions. Outlined below are the characteristics frequently attributed to the various kinds of objections found in the literature.

Medical exemptions

Medical exemptions were once considered the most concrete of all the exemption categories and generated little debate. Recently, however, medical exemptions have become more controversial, given the perceived ease with which they are granted. Gostin (2005) provides a solid interpretation of medical exemptions: specifically, individuals with compromised immune systems or other physical conditions, such as allergies, that increase the risk of vaccine-induced injuries are exempt from immunisation. Medical exemptions are typically accompanied by a letter from a healthcare provider and in the past have been accepted unconditionally (Salmon et al, 2006). Individuals with medical contraindications for vaccination rely on herd immunity to protect them from vaccine-preventable diseases (Bradley, 1999; Wynia, 2007a).

Religious exemptions

Religious objections, a sub-category of non-medical conscientious objections to vaccination, are typically recognised as grounds for exemption. In the US, all but two states, West Virginia and Mississippi, permit religious exemptions (Salmon et al, 2004; Salmon et al, 2005). As early as 1798, vaccination was perceived by many individuals as "meddling in the work of God" (Abbey, 2002, p 1717). Even today, some individuals in developed and developing countries maintain that immunisation programmes challenge God's predetermined plan and that complying with state vaccination mandates is therefore unconscionable (Spier, 2002).

Individuals may also seek religious exemption from vaccination because a handful of the vaccines on the market stem from aborted foetal cell strains (Zimmerman, 2004; Salmon et al, 2005). However, some religious leaders and theologians specialising in ethics have outlined explanations as to why vaccinations, even those made from aborted foetal cell lines, tissues and/or blood, are not antithetical to certain religious beliefs (Grabenstein, 2003; Pontificia Academia Pro Vita, 2005). Several ethicists at the National Catholic Bioethics Center and elsewhere considered the virology, epidemiology and theology of the matter in detail. They concluded that the association between implicated vaccines and abortion was non complicit, and that using these vaccines is not contrary to a principled opposition to abortion (Grabenstein, 2003, p 1338).

Some theologians have provided ethical arguments, permitting vaccination within certain faiths. However, the extent to which such religious views are known, understood and/or shared by adherents is unknown, especially considering that individuals can decide against vaccination for religious reasons without providing a signature from a religious leader, thus increasing the likelihood that religious counselling did not occur (Salmon and Siegel, 2001). Moreover, there is an apparent paucity of accessible information with respect to different religious traditions' positions on immunisation, which can significantly impede individuals as they endeavour to make sound health decisions for themselves and/or their families.

Philosophical exemptions

Prior to the possibility of objecting to vaccination on philosophical grounds, many individuals opposed to vaccination claimed religious exemption (Salmon et al, 2005). However, permitting religious exemptions only was deemed unconstitutional and, consequently, philosophical objections emerged as a legitimate exemption possibility (Salmon and Siegel, 2001). Today, 19 states of the US allow philosophical exemptions (Salmon et al, 2004; 2005). Philosophical rationales used to support exemption include, as previously mentioned, the compulsory nature of vaccination and the perceived inappropriate role of the state interfering in the private lives of individuals and their families (Arnup, 1992; Colgrove, 2005; Blume, 2006). Other philosophical objections, not unlike religious concerns, derive from ethical concerns about the creation of the vaccines themselves, such as the use of aborted foetal cell strains, tissue and blood, and animal testing (Colgrove, 2005; Salmon et al, 2005). Opponents of immunisation have also claimed philosophical exemption based on divergent views regarding how healthcare resources are spent: specifically, vaccination programmes rather than improved nutrition, sanitation and hygiene (Arnup, 1992). Alternative medicine practitioners such as homeopaths and chiropractors, in addition to proponents of the "physical culture" (Colgrove, 2005, p 178) and "broader popular health movement" (Arnup, 1992, p 169), were among the individuals claiming philosophical objections to vaccination in a demonstration of resistance against the "hegemony of allopathic practice" (Colgrove, 2005, p 177).

Personal exemptions

In the developed world, the incidence rate of vaccine-preventable diseases has diminished so significantly that the fear of vaccine-induced illness now outweighs (at least for some people) the risks of contracting the illness without vaccination (Bradley, 1999; Spier, 2002; Ulmer and Liu, 2002; Verweij and Dawson, 2004; Blume, 2006). The rare adverse events resulting from vaccinations are publicised extensively in the media, without reference to the numbers of vaccine success stories, which contributes to public fear and anxiety (Spier, 2002; Fair et al, 2002). Consequently, increasing numbers of individuals are refusing vaccines/seeking exemptions based on concerns surrounding vaccine safety (Salmon et al, 2005; Blume, 2006). Vaccination refusals (particularly on behalf of children) because of perceived risks and health concerns are sometimes categorised as philosophical or conscientious objections (Colgrove, 2005; Blume, 2006). Although drawing a connection between safety and the 'do no harm' philosophical principle is not difficult (Wicclair, 2000), one might argue that the crux of an individual refusal is more basic, rooted in the vaccine itself and the potentially disastrous consequences of an adverse effect. One might argue that individual fears and anxieties are not 'philosophical' in and of themselves, but rather are a reaction to news media, experiences of friends and family, and a failure on the part of public health officials to acknowledge and validate those fears and work to assuage them.

Colgrove (2005) acknowledges that objecting to vaccination on the basis of concerns surrounding the vaccination itself is not equivalent to a philosophical objection:

> Far greater were the numbers of ordinary citizens who opposed the practice not because of philosophical principles but because they objected to the discomfort and inconvenience [of the vaccine]. (p 180)

Clearly, new descriptors are necessary to explain exemptions based on concerns surrounding vaccine safety and discomfort. The terms 'personal' (Salmon and Siegel, 2001; Salmon et al, 2006) and 'conscientious' (Blume, 2006), seemingly adopted to capture the nuances of such objections, arguably indicate the grey area that exists when addressing philosophical objections to immunisation.

The adjective 'personal' acknowledges that philosophical exemptions do not accurately convey all of the reasons why individuals object to vaccination. For instance, seeking exemption on the basis of fears associated with vaccine safety and/or health repercussions is a personal reason. Personal objections also represent a larger, systemic challenge faced by public health departments – namely the combined need to educate the public about the benefits and risks of vaccination and to continue to pursue safe and effective vaccines. Specifically, the perceived threat of vaccine-preventable diseases has diminished and, consequently, the fear of vaccines has increased. As the direct risk of vaccine-preventable infection diminishes, the more the state asks individuals to assume the risk of vaccination that increases in relationship to the actual risk of the disease. Therefore, the state has a duty of reciprocity (that is, no-fault compensation) to care for individuals whose health has been compromised as a result of vaccines, especially in regions where vaccination programmes are mandatory. Exemptions based on concerns surrounding vaccine safety and/or individual misconceptions about the likeliness of contracting the illness without the vaccine, and the degree to which the vaccine-preventable disease is 'dangerous' (Salmon et al, 2005) represent more than personal objections. Rather, such rationales are arguably demonstrative of public health's lapse in health education and an accompanying sense of resignation, an acceptance that some people will simply refuse vaccines.

Similarly, other reasons reported among the different requests for exemption (categorised as personal exemptions) have to do with societal barriers such as "poor access or non-availability of vaccination" (Bradley, 1999, p 332) rather than a genuine aversion towards immunisation (Bradley, 1999; Salmon et al, 1999; Salmon and Siegel, 2001; McIntyre et al, 2003). Such reasons for opting out pertain to the vaccination process and associated employment challenges, specifically the unpaid time missed from work that can result from immunisation (Colgrove, 2005; Wynia, 2007b). Surprisingly, such exemptions have been defined, or perhaps more accurately dismissed, as personal objections, and no appeals have been made to public health departments to fulfil their obligations to the community, particularly its marginalised members. It is these exemptions that are now categorised and introduced here as social barrier exemptions.

Proposed efforts to reduce vaccination exemptions: create review boards

The variety of exemption claims to which individuals can appeal, coupled with the perceived ease with which vaccination exemptions are granted, led Salmon and colleagues (Salmon et al, 1999; Salmon and Siegel, 2001; Salmon and Omer, 2006; Salmon et al, 2006), as well as other scholars addressing the issue of the role of conscientious objection in medicine (Card, 2007; LaFollette, 2007; Meyers and Woods, 2007; Richman, 2007; Wicclair, 2007a; 2007b), to question whether a mechanism should be implemented in the US to assess the sincerity of the individual's claim rather than questioning the belief itself. Salmon and colleagues (2006) appear to disapprove of the ease with which exemptions are granted, because the higher the exemption rate the lower the herd immunity, which purportedly leads to an increased likelihood of disease outbreaks, thus rendering compulsory vaccination programmes ineffective. Salmon and Siegel (2001) note that filing for religious or philosophical exemptions requires less effort than completing the vaccination requirements – most individuals just need to sign a form and never interact with a healthcare provider – and the "ease of obtaining an exemption has been quantitatively associated with the frequency of exemptions" (p 290). Some states require individuals seeking religious exemption to produce a confirmatory letter from their religious leader, whereas others simply require a signed form (Salmon and Siegel, 2001). Salmon and Siegel (2001) suggest that minimising the focus currently spent on the nature of objections and focusing instead on implementing a more stringent process of exemption (such as individual education counselling sessions) would serve to prove an individual's opposition to vaccination and be more effective in decreasing exemption rates, as it would eliminate the possibility of an 'easy' or 'lazy' way out.

One problem, however, with not focusing on the nature of the exemption request removes any remaining checks and balances that exist in public health. Specifically, individuals 'objecting' to vaccination because they do not have access to vaccines or cannot afford the process (for example, the cost of the vaccine, transport to the clinic, time off work, potential illness) is important information for public health officials to know, as it suggests that new strategic approaches are necessary for effective and efficient vaccination campaigns. Similarly, if individuals request personal exemptions because they have incorrect or only partial information about the benefits and risks of vaccination, then exemption decisions are not truly informed and reflect weaknesses in public health education. Preserving a transparent exemption process also signals to religious leaders that increased focus on medical ethics as it pertains to their respective religions is necessary. As science and technology advance, new ethical issues emerge and many patients want religious guidance in their healthcare decision making. For example, if individuals seek religious exemption because of the use of foetal cell lines in select vaccines, yet religious officials have concluded that such vaccinations are not contrary to the faith, a sizeable number of non-vaccinated individuals might have made different decisions had they been privy to accurate religious information.

Moreover, one might argue that the money that would be required to enable individual educational counselling for potential conscientious objectors would be better spent in assisting individuals who are willing to be vaccinated but do not have the financial means or resources to do so, or those who, according to Salmon et al (2006), are just "lazy or indifferent" (p 437). For example, providing assistance such as home vaccinations, education sessions and arrangements with workplaces to provide compensation for sick days resulting from immunisation could positively influence vaccination uptake. Of course, education is an important part of healthcare decision making and, given the increasing number of conscientious objections (Salmon and Siegel, 2001), vaccine education should arguably be conveniently available to all individuals, not just those threatening exemption. Perhaps such informational sessions could occur during annual health check-ups or during prenatal sessions, so as to minimise the number of trips to the clinic or hospital.

Finally, increasing the difficulty of obtaining exemptions by requiring educational sessions cannot possibly shed light on the strength of an individual's religious, philosophical, personal or conscience-based convictions, although it may serve as a deterrent for the 'lazy'. If individuals have the time and money available to defend their beliefs in educational sessions, who would be responsible for deciding whether an individual was "honestly opposed" (Salmon et al, 2006, p 437), and on what grounds would those decisions be based? In a society that has legally upheld the fundamental right of "bodily self-determination" (Berkeley, 2005, p 40) and imposed limits on state interventions with respect to "privacy, freedom of association, and individual liberties" (Gostin, 2004, p 572), how can governments request permission to judge individual beliefs? Moreover, creating obstacles to vaccine exemption for individuals conceivably only increases costs for people whose reasons for exempting initially may have had to do with limited resources. Such stringent exemption policies may also force individuals with strong objections to vaccines to get vaccinated because of the severe cost in time and money to prove their convictions – luxuries that not all members of society possess. In a sense, imposing additional mandates and barriers on citizens is the equivalent of implementing a process that further marginalises individuals while simultaneously violating their human rights and, ultimately, their health.

Freedom of conscience: an inalienable human right?

To implement a public health vaccination programme that respects and protects human rights as outlined in the UDHR (United Nations, 1948) requires an improved understanding of the term 'conscience'. Despite the history of conscience and its development as a concept over the centuries, some contemporary theorists maintain that conscience does not exist (Langston, 2001). However, the authors of the UDHR (United Nations, 1948) scripted a secular use of conscience into the document three times: in the preamble, in Article 1 and in Article 18.

In addition, conscience is similarly mentioned in the Siracusa Principles (ECOSOC, 1984), a non-ratified document that outlines certain principles that should be non-derogable, even if the state is threatened. Among these principles is freedom of conscience:

> No state party shall, even in time of emergency threatening the life of the nation, derogate from the Covenant's guarantees of the right to life; freedom from torture, cruel, inhuman or degrading treatment or punishment, and from medical or scientific experimentation without free consent … and freedom of thought, conscience and religion. These are not derogable under any conditions even for the asserted purpose of preserving the life of the nation. (Section II, Part D, No 58)

How are individuals and governments meant to interpret conscience?

Under Article 18 of the UDHR (United Nations, 1948) conscience is underscored as unique and separate from freedom of thought and freedom of religion. Langston (2001) argues that conscience is often used in everyday language to capture more elaborate, complex phrases. Is the secular use of the word 'conscience' in the UDHR a popular use of the term that flows well with thought and religion? Is there a presumed shared, global understanding of the meaning of conscience? Are such assumptions wise, given the complexity of conscience and the ongoing philosophical debates surrounding its nature and ultimate existence? Langston (2001) mentions the possibility of using "the term *conscience* with a background of public agreement about its definitions and application without assuming that there is such an entity" (p 107). What was the public agreement surrounding the definition of conscience when the UDHR (United Nations, 1948) was crafted?

Is understanding 'conscience' as used in the UDHR (United Nations, 1948) integral to forming public health vaccination programmes that protect human rights and enable individuals to make legitimate (not coerced) personal decisions that may include refusing vaccines? Was the ambiguous use of 'conscience' intentional in that it can be defined differently for people depending on their individual circumstances? Does 'conscience' even need a definition and do individuals need to explain why they evoke the 'freedom of conscience' clause? Is refusing to be vaccinated for reasons of conscience sufficient without an explanation and, if so, does that change how we perceive other non-medical exemption typologies, such as philosophical, personal and religious exemptions? Do conscience-based objections even need an explanation? If they do not, are there consequences for individual and population health and does it matter if there are?

Conclusion: public health, human rights and vaccination

Public health and human rights are united in their interest in identifying social determinants of health, as social determinants underscore human rights violations which affect the health of individuals and, by extension, the population (Mann et al, 1999; Colgrove and Bayer, 2005). A growing body of evidence supports the argument that health policies that protect human rights ultimately foster population health (Mann et al, 1999; Colgrove and Bayer, 2005; Mariner et al, 2005; Wynia, 2005). Vaccination programmes, like other population health initiatives, have not managed to escape the social barriers to health (Bradley, 1999; Salmon et al, 1999; Salmon and Siegel, 2001; McIntyre et al, 2003). Unfortunately, the vaccination literature has not focused on the existing social inequities when evaluating the successes and failures of national and international immunisation efforts in developed countries. Such neglect is due, in part, to the language used to discuss vaccination programmes and those individuals who choose not to get vaccinated. Although some individuals are conscientious objectors seeking exemption for religious, philosophical, personal or conscience-based reasons, evidence suggests that others seek exemption because social barriers prevent them from partaking in publicly endorsed preventive health measures. However, rather than engaging in efforts to minimise the marginalisation of certain populations and individuals, public health discussions tend to focus on introducing or reinforcing compulsory vaccination programmes as possible solutions to counteract increasing rates of philosophical and personal objections.

As articulated throughout this chapter, significant drawbacks often accompany compulsory vaccination programmes, leading to uptake outcomes contrary to those intended. Goals that public health departments can achieve through voluntary public participation are preferable to those achieved through coercive or intrusive measures. Given the effects of herd immunity, the low incidence of vaccine-preventable diseases and the overall support for vaccination programmes, the risk of infection from non-immunised individuals to immunised individuals is low. Therefore, Bradley (1999) encourages individuals concerned about falling ill to vaccine-preventable diseases to get themselves immunised rather than incite governments to impose compulsory vaccination programmes on an entire society.

As public health authorities consider strategies for increasing the numbers of adults who get vaccinated, a critical look at the existing strategies implemented in immunisation programmes is required, along with consideration of the adjustments that public health programmes can make to improve uptake without further limiting individual rights. Recognising how vaccine language serves to conceal potential weaknesses in existing programmes not only is a disservice to programmes and taxpayers but also compromises individual and public health. Failing to ensure that all individuals who want vaccines – or who would want vaccines if they had a better understanding of the risks and benefits – receive them is a direct violation of human rights, specifically, the right to health. Consequently, programme redesign efforts are necessary to preserve individual and population health.

As public health departments around the world face the arrival of new health challenges, such as pandemic influenza, gaining and keeping the public's trust will be essential for new vaccination programmes to work and existing programmes to be sustained (Verweij and Dawson, 2004; Gostin, 2004; Salmon et al, 2005; Blume, 2006). Too often, public health authorities minimise the risks associated with health initiatives and interventions. Over time, health risks emerge and the repercussions of losing trust within the community are significant (Blume, 2006). As countries consider new vaccine programmes for future epidemics and pandemics, public health officials should remember that public concerns surrounding vaccine safety are not completely irrational, as mass immunisation initiatives can fail (as evidenced in 1976 with the US swine flu epidemic, Gostin, 2004). Most importantly, adopting a language for exemptions that more accurately reflects systemic barriers in the vaccination process for certain members of society, rather than using catchphrases that burden, and in many respects blame, the individual objector, is crucial.

Additional readings

Gostin, L. (2005) '*Jacobson v Massachusetts* at 100 years: police power and civil liberties in tension', *American Journal of Public Health*, vol 95, no 4, pp 576–80.

Langston, D. (2001) *Conscience and other virtues*, Pennsylvania: Pennsylvania State University Press.

Mann, J., Gruskin S., Grodin M. and Annas G. (eds) (1999) *Health and human rights*, New York: Routledge.

References

Abbey, D. (2002) 'Anti-vaccination web sites', *Journal of the American Medical Association*, vol 288, no 14, p 1717.

Arnup, K. (1992) '"Victims of vaccination?": opposition to compulsory immunization in Ontario, 1900–90', *Canadian Bulletin of Medical History*, vol 9, no 2, pp 159–76.

Berkeley, R. (2005) 'When medicine and religion collide: court rulings provide guidance on dealing with this thorny issue', *Medical Economics*, vol 82, no 17, pp 40–4.

Blume, S. (2006) 'Anti-vaccination movements and their interpretations', *Social Science and Medicine*, vol 62, pp 628–42.

Bradley, P. (1999) 'Should childhood immunisation be compulsory?', *Journal of Medical Ethics*, vol 25, no 4, pp 330–34.

Card, R. (2007) 'Conscientious objection and emergency contraception', *The American Journal of Bioethics*, vol 7, no 6, pp 8–14.

Colgrove, J. (2005) '"Science in a democracy": the contested status of vaccination in the progressive era and the 1920s', *Isis*, vol 96, no 2, pp 167–91.

Colgrove, J. and Bayer, R. (2005) 'Manifold restraints: liberty, public health, and the legacy of *Jacobson v Massachusetts*', *American Journal of Public Health*, vol 95, no 4, pp 571–6.

ECOSOC (United Nations Economic and Social Council), UN Sub-commission on Prevention of Discrimination and Protection of Minorities (1984) *Siracusa Principles on the Limitation and Derogation of Provisions in the International Covenant on Civil and Political Rights, Annex, UN Doc E/CN.4/1984/4*. Available at: http://hei.unige.ch/~clapham/hrdoc/docs/siracusa.html (accessed 14 January 2007).

Fair, E., Murphy, T., Golaz, A. and Wharton, M. (2002) 'Philosophic objection to vaccination as a risk for tetanus among children younger than 15 years', *Pediatrics*, vol 109, no 1, p E2.

Gostin, L. (2004) 'Pandemic influenza: public health preparedness for the next global health emergency', *The Journal of Law, Medicine & Ethics*, vol 32, no 4, pp 565–73.

Gostin, L. (2005) 'Jacobson v Massachusetts at 100 years: police power and civil liberties in tension', *American Journal of Public Health*, vol 95, no 4, pp 576–80.

Grabenstein, J. (2003) 'Where medicine and religion intersect', *The Annals of Pharmacotherapy*, vol 37, no 9, pp 1338–9.

LaFollette, H. (2007) 'The physician's conscience', *The American Journal of Bioethics*, vol 7, no 12, pp 15–17.

Langston, D. (2001) *Conscience and other virtues*, Pennsylvania: The Pennsylvania State University Press.

Lawrence, R. and Curlin, F. (2007) 'Clash of definitions: controversies about conscience in medicine and open peer commentary', *The American Journal of Bioethics*, vol 7, no 12, pp 10–34.

Mann, J., Gostin, L., Gruskin, S., Brennan, T., Lazzarini, Z. and Fineberg, H. (1999) 'Health and human rights', in J. Mann, S. Gruskin, M. Grodin and G. Annas (eds) *Health and human rights*, New York: Routledge.

Mariner, W., Annas, G. and Glantz, L. (2005) '*Jacobson v Massachusetts*: it's not your great-great-grandfather's public health law', *American Journal of Public Health*, vol 95, no 4, pp 581–90.

McIntyre, P., Williams, A. and Leask, J. (2003) 'Refusal of parents to vaccinate: dereliction of duty or legitimate personal choice?' *The Medical Journal of Australia*, vol 178, no 4, pp 150–1.

Meyers, C. and Woods, R. (2007) 'Conscientious objection? Yes, but make sure it is genuine', *The American Journal of Bioethics*, vol 7, no 6, pp 19–21.

Pontificia Academia Pro Vita (2005) 'Moral reflections on vaccines prepared from cells derived from aborted human foetuses', *The National Catholic Bioethics Quarterly*, vol 6, no 3, pp 541–7.

Richman, K. (2007) 'Pharmacists and the social contract', *The American Journal of Bioethics*, vol 7, no 6, pp 15–16.

Salmon, D. and Omer, S. (2006) 'Individual freedoms versus collective responsibility: immunization decision-making in the face of occasionally competing values', *Emerging Themes in Epidemiology*, vol 3, no 13. Available at: www.ete-online.com/content/3/1/13 (accessed 27 August 2008).

Salmon, D. and Siegel, A. (2001) 'Religious and philosophical exemptions from vaccination requirements and lessons learned from conscientious objectors from conscription', *Public Health Reports*, vol 116, no 4, pp 289–95.

Salmon, D., Haber, M., Gangarosa, E., Phillips, L., Smith, N. and Chen, R. (1999) 'Health consequences of religious and philosophical exemptions from immunization laws', *Journal of the American Medical Association*, vol 281, no 1, pp 47–53.

Salmon, D., Moulton, L., Omer, S., Chace, L., Klassen, A., Talebian, P. and Halsey, N. (2004) 'Knowledge, attitudes, and beliefs of school nurses and personnel and associations with nonmedical immunization exemptions', *Pediatrics*, vol 113, no 6, pp 552–9.

Salmon, D., Moulton, L., Omer, S., de Hart, M., Stokley, S. and Halsey, N. (2005) 'Factors associated with refusal of childhood vaccines among parents of school-aged children', *Archives of Pediatrics and Adolescent Medicine*, vol 159, no 5, pp 470–6.

Salmon, D., Teret, S., MacIntyre, C., Salisbury, D., Burgess, M. and Halsey, N. (2006) 'Compulsory vaccination and conscientious or philosophical exemptions: past, present, and future', *The Lancet*, vol 367, no 9508, pp 436–42.

Spier, R. (2002) 'Perception of risk of vaccine adverse events: a historical perspective', *Vaccine*, vol 20, pp S78–S84.

Ulmer, J. and Liu, M. (2002) 'Ethical issues for vaccines and immunisation', *Nature Reviews Immunology*, vol 2, no 4, pp 291–6.

United Nations (1948) *Universal Declaration of Human Rights*. Adopted and proclaimed by UN General Assembly Resolution 217A(III) (10 December 1948). Available at www.un.org/Overview/rights.html (accessed 14 January 2007).

Verweij, M. and Dawson, A. (2004) 'Ethical principles for collective immunisation programmes', *Vaccine*, vol 22, no 23–24, pp 3122–6.

Wicclair, M. (2000) 'Conscientious objection in medicine', *Bioethics*, vol 14, no 3, pp 205–27.

Wicclair, M. (2007a) 'Reasons and healthcare professionals' claims of conscience', *The American Journal of Bioethics*, vol 7, no 6, pp 21–2.

Wicclair, M. (2007b) 'The moral significance of claims of conscience in healthcare', *The American Journal of Bioethics*, vol 7, no 12, pp 30–31.

Wynia, M. (2005) 'Oversimplifications II: public health ethics ignores individual rights', *The American Journal of Bioethics*, vol 5, no 5, pp 6–8.

Wynia, M. (2007a) 'Mandating vaccination: what counts as a "mandate" in public health and when should they be used?', *The American Journal of Bioethics*, vol 7, no 12, pp 2–6.

Wynia, M. (2007b) 'Ethics and public health emergencies: restrictions on liberty', *The American Journal of Bioethics*, vol 7, no 2, pp 1–5.

Zimmerman, R. (2004) 'Ethical analyses of vaccines grown in human cell strains derived from abortion: arguments and internet search', *Vaccine*, vol 22, no 31–32, pp 4238–44.

Part Three
Public health ethics: developing
a basis for practice

TWELVE

Theory and practice in public health ethics: a complex relationship

Angus Dawson

It is an exciting time in the nascent field of public health ethics. This feeling seems to exist among those approaching these issues from a more theoretical perspective as well as those with a more practical or practitioner point of view. The thing that unites us is a sense that there is something missing from traditional medical ethics. This feeling may in turn be explained in three possible ways. First, many topics central to public health are missing from the list of issues tackled in mainstream medical ethics. Second, there is concern about the adequacy of the theoretical approach or assumptions that have been used in medical ethics once they are applied to examples in public health. Or, third, both of these may be true. The danger is that while we can agree that we are involved in a common project, it remains the case that we have different aims, languages and priorities, and the opportunity for genuine communication and collaboration is missed.[1]

This chapter is a preliminary exploration of some of the issues that arise as we attempt to bring these different perspectives together. It is common to use the metaphor of a 'gap' between theory and practice when trying to articulate this problem. I choose not to do so, because I think it both overestimates and underestimates the problem. It overestimates because the very best work in applied ethics is both theoretically rigorous (or at least defensible) and of practical importance. It underestimates the problem because we do not just have two clear camps (the 'theorists' and the 'practitioners'). Even if it makes sense to think of them as distinct groups, no unity exists in either category. Theorists (in the sense intended) will include philosophers from different schools (realist, pragmatist, postmodern and so on) and advocates of different normative theories (consequentialism, deontology, virtue theory and others), but will also include perspectives from other disciplines (psychology, communication studies, sociology, anthropology, history, political sciences and so on). The practitioners are also a diverse bunch (and will include front-line public health physicians and nurses, dieticians, politicians, policy advisors, health promoters, charities, environmental scientists, food inspectors, water engineers, dentists and others). As a result it is hardly a surprise that the relationship between theory and practice is a complex one. It is less of a 'gap' than a huge continent, full of diverse habitats, microclimates and populations. If we are to provide any coherent understanding of this complex landmass we need, urgently, to seek ways to facilitate genuine dialogue among the diverse inhabitants.[2]

In this chapter I attempt to offer some help in sketching a map to aid such future exploration and discussion. I focus on three related core ideas. First, I outline and discuss the relationship between three related but distinct concepts: 'theories', 'frameworks' and 'models'. Second, I focus in some detail on a discussion of frameworks, because I see them as being the most plausible means of drawing together insights from the theoretical and the practical. In doing so I discuss some recent literature about frameworks as a means of suggesting what they are, what their focus ought to be, and what constraints we should place upon them. Third, I turn to what I see as a key assumption that underlies much recent discussion of public health ethics – that priority should be given to individual liberty. This assumption is understandable, given the way that discussion in public health ethics has drawn on the existing theoretical insights of medical ethics, but I argue that it is mistaken. Instead, I suggest that we ought to embrace a view of public health ethics that derives from the nature of public health itself, one that sees a more interventionist role for the state in protecting and promoting the health of the public. This seems to be deeply unfashionable, but I will argue that it is the only defensible position if we are to take public health (in either a theoretical or a practical sense) seriously.

Theories, frameworks and models: a rough taxonomy

In this section I want to explore the meaning of, and relationship between, three related concepts: theory, framework and model. These terms are often used interchangeably. While I don't believe that any of these concepts ultimately has especially clear boundaries, I think we can still distinguish key differences which mean that the core element of each concept can be seen to be distinct from the other two. I think it makes sense to identify the central element of each concept with a particular role. However, I accept that this is not clear cut and each of the three concepts may contain aspects of each of the three different roles I identify.

I begin with what we mean when we talk of a theory. I take a **theory** (at least in the sense of a normative moral theory) to be primarily interested in the *justification* of action (through the suggestion of reasons why a proposed or completed action was right or wrong, or what we ought to do and why this is the case). Examples of such theories might include consequentialist, deontological or egalitarian views, justified through arguments over the rights and wrongs of substantive normative moral or political theory. Second, I take a **framework** to be primarily interested in providing some context for or assistance with *deliberation* about what we ought to do in a particular context. Although a framework ought ultimately to be linked in a clear way with theory and questions of justification, a framework is, as it were, 'closer' to the reality of day-to-day decision making in an applied context. In this sense, there is nothing wrong with a framework taking certain theoretical considerations for granted and concentrating upon aiding busy decision makers through the provision of a checklist of relevant considerations, principles and issues to keep in mind. Frameworks will generally be pragmatic and ought to be focused on aiding the performance of appropriate actions. (I will say far more about frameworks in the next section.) Third, I take the primary role of models to be one of *explanation*. A **model** helps us to understand the world around us, by offering a deliberately simplified or perspectival view of a problem or issue. A model may use a guiding metaphor or diagram to help us understand an aspect of the world.[3] So I think that frameworks and models have, to borrow an analogy from the philosophy of mind, different primary directions of fit. A framework aids us in *acting upon* the world, whereas as a model helps us to *understand* it.[4] So if this approach is correct, we end up with a rough taxonomy like this:

Concept	Primary role
Theory	Justification
Framework	Deliberation
Model	Explanation

I repeat my note of caution: this taxonomy only provides the *primary* role for each of these three concepts. I am not suggesting that there is any exclusive and neat one-to-one mapping of each concept to each role. Nevertheless, I think there is something in the idea that we should keep these roles in mind as we think about which of these three particular concepts might be most useful to us on a particular occasion.[5] I will say nothing further about models in this chapter. In the next section I will discuss the idea of frameworks in some depth, but for the rest of this section I will say a little about theories and their role in public health ethics.

I have suggested that the main role of a normative moral theory is to provide coherent justifications for our actions. Of course, which particular theory we ought to adopt will in turn be subject to vigorous debate. I will leave this issue to one side, to be settled on another occasion. I don't actually think it is the most pressing issue, as very often different theoretical positions provide very similar answers, even if the reasons for those answers might differ. I will focus here on a different issue: where ought we to start when we think about adopting or evaluating an adequate theory for the relevant domain of discourse that we have in mind (in this case, public health)? There is a strong tendency to think that we ought to start with theory. In this view, even within an interdisciplinary approach, the philosophical task is held to be *preliminary* to other activities: the key is to sort out the theory before we move on to the domain of application.

There are a number of problems with this 'theory first' approach, not the least of which will be the eternal wait for the philosophers to settle their differences about the appropriate moral theory to use. However, perhaps more directly pressing in this case is a general problem of theory formation: that is, what kind of conditions of relevance can we apply if we do not have a particular domain of activity in mind (such as public health) as we develop our theory in the first place? We may produce a perfect and beautiful theory, which unfortunately is completely irrelevant when it comes to answering the kinds of issues to be faced in the real world. On the other hand, a focus on pure practice (immune from any theoretical assumptions) upon which we attempt to 'build up' to our theory also looks problematic. Here the worry is that the resultant 'theory' is just a formalised version of existing practice, with little real normative *bite*. The standard contemporary answer to this dilemma is to invoke some form of reflective equilibrium: an active moderating movement back and forth between theory and cases or individual judgements.[6] However, I also have some reservations about this kind of appeal to a coherentist methodology.[7] I prefer to think that the best way to make progress in developing a practice-related theory is to specify a domain of activity such as public health, explore the aims and activities which are at its core, and then use this to (provisionally) explore more theoretical perspectives upon the issues concerned.

On this view, it is public health as a type of practice that constrains the production of an appropriate normative theory: thinking what public health ethics ought to be must begin by looking to see what happens in public health.[8] This does not mean endorsing everything that goes on in the name of promoting public health, but it does mean taking care to ensure that we don't simply reject everything with that motivation as morally wrong. Once we have some idea of what happens in public health we can begin to formulate a clear concept of what 'public health' is, and then in turn use this as a central element in determining the limits to an adequate normative theory of public health ethics; one that can be used in public health practice. So, on this approach, public health ethics is to a large extent motivated and justified in terms of thinking about public health as a special type of social activity, with a clear focus on a particular set of aims (such as improving population welfare, reducing inequalities, reducing or removing harms and so on), methods (such as epidemiology, social survey tools and so on), actions (for example, interventions through the law, education, information, taxation and others) and outcomes (such as removing harms, improving quality of life, promoting equity and so on). In other words, a conception of public health ought to be the foundation for public health ethics. Such an approach will provide us with the best way of finding our way around the complex continent upon which we stand.

Frameworks: aims, tasks and limits

I turn now to a discussion of frameworks. What is a framework? What job do they do? What job ought they to do? One of the reasons why a discussion of frameworks may be useful is because of the diversity of ways in which people define this term. For example, a 'framework' is often used as a description for a set of values or principles that have been placed at the beginning of a policy document produced by a committee mandated to formulate a policy on a particular issue or narrow set of issues. Here, the framework may be a general expression of the values that have influenced the deliberations of the committee, or it may have a stronger role than this as generative or determinative (in some sense) of the policy conclusions. It is this kind of framework that Giacomini et al (2009) are most interested in exploring in their discussion of the use of frameworks in Canadian policy documents.[9] Second, there will be cases where there is no obvious link between a framework and a policy (even where they are side-by-side in a policy document). Here what is called a 'framework' is a general expression of the kind of values that the committee is committed to (or the ones that they tend to like or dislike). The danger is that this just results in 'boo/hurray' policy making, with no clear link between the policy advocated and the value statements made. Third, other uses of the term 'framework' tend to refer to a more general set of principles that can be applied to individual cases (for example, the four principles might be seen as a framework in this sense).[10] However, as I suggested above, I see the primary role of a framework as being to aid deliberation by making relevant values explicit. These values are then used to guide or 'frame' decision making. They may well be formulated at the level of a general area of discourse (such as public health) or they may be specific to a particular problem (for example, mass preventive vaccination). It is important, then, to see core cases of frameworks as merely 'framing devices'. In other words, it makes no sense to criticise any framework for failing to contain well worked-out, substantive, theoretically justified answers to deep, normative questions. If it focuses on such things, it ceases to be a framework and adopts more of a theoretical role, as its primary intent becomes one of offering a justified account for the answers provided.

So, in my view the relationship between frameworks and theoretical entities such as moral theories is a complex one, but we ought generally to try to keep the two entities separate. There will be a relationship between the two, but there is no reason to think it will be a direct deductive one, with theory being *prior* or *superior* to a framework. They just perform different tasks. Frameworks ought to be flexible, relatively general, pragmatic and orientated towards action. So, I disagree with Holland's view (Chapter Three) when, in his discussion of frameworks, he says: "Frameworks suggest rigid constructions into which can be shoehorned the discussion of any public health ethics problem" (pp 39–40). If a framework is 'rigid' in this sense it is not a framework, but more like a theory. Holland distinguishes what he calls frameworks from principled approaches and he holds the latter to be superior. However, in his discussion of frameworks he includes both what I think of as a paradigm case of a framework (Kass, 2001) and what I think of as a paradigm case of a principled approach to public health ethics (Childress et al, 2002). Holland focuses on the diversity of ethical challenges that emerge in public health and asks, rhetorically, "Is it really feasible to think that all these can be fitted into one framework?" (p 40). Of course, there is no reason to assume there will be one framework for public health, as frameworks might be based around different problems, issues, or areas of practice and so on. But even if we assume that there will be only one framework, I don't see why principled approaches to public health ethics do not have the same problem that he suggests characterise frameworks, only multiplied. The kind of thing he means by a 'principled' approach is actually a type of theoretical approach: the principles are justified prior to and independently of the context within which they are applied. This is actually more rigid and allows for far less flexibility than a framework (in my sense).

So, let's leave the issue of the definition of a framework to one side and switch to thinking about the kinds of condition or limit that we want to place on the use of frameworks. A good place to start is with the discussion in Giacomini et al (2009). This article makes some good points with regard to the role of frameworks in general. For example, they stress the need for coherence both internally (the various elements must fit together in an appropriate way) and externally (the framework itself must tie up in an appropriate way to the recommended policy outcomes). I also think it is helpful to make clear the need to distinguish different possible elements of a framework (for example, goals for a policy are different from both the procedural values that apply in the application of a policy and the substantive values that may justify or inform the policy). These very different things are often confused and presented all together in one framework.[11] There are various problems with any such mixed approach, but the main one is that it becomes very unclear how these different elements relate to each other. Can procedural values be 'weighed' or 'traded' against substantive values, or are they incompatible in some sense because they have a different status? Presumably the aims of a framework need to be determined before the framework itself is formulated, and they must link up with the aims of the policy intervention that is the subject of the framework.

However, I think there are some questionable assumptions behind Giacomini et al's (2009) critique. For example, they devote a large part of their article to focusing on disagreement in the diverse range of ethical frameworks that they review. On the face of it, this seems to be an odd complaint. Why should we think there must be a single framework to cover all policy cases? Arguably, the ethical issues relating to biotechnology and infectious disease have little in common, so I don't see why we should expect there to be a shared framework covering both cases. Or to give another of their examples, it seems appropriate for a health technology assessment framework to contain a value such as "[i]nnovation should be encouraged and supported" (p 62), but it is not clear that this is so relevant to infectious disease control.

Where, of course, it may make sense to have just one approach is when we switch to talking about theories and the justification of actions. However, interestingly, Giacomini et al seem happy to accept disagreement and a certain relativism at the level of theory. They suggest that a framework can act as a solution to this problem, as follows: "Value conflicts are inevitable, and ethical frameworks promise a shared language and focus for consensus building" (2009, p 66).[12] Presumably, they mean that even though we may be relativists at the meta-ethical level we may still accept an agreed framework. However, I am not clear how this view sits with their prior complaint about the diversity of frameworks. They also seem concerned about the fact that there is no agreement on the meaning of key concepts such as 'transparency' and 'equity' in the various frameworks they explore. Again, it seems natural that such diversity does exist, given the disagreement apparent in discussion of such normative concepts. However, this implies nothing about the true normative status of these concepts, nor does the mere fact of disagreement over the meaning of such concepts entail the conclusion that we cannot agree on a theory or a framework. Giacomini et al's positive suggestions, in the end, seem relatively weak, in that they propose a set of procedural values as a solution to the problems they present (2009, pp 66, 67).[13]

Perhaps it will help to further the discussion if we consider a particular framework in some detail.[14] Possibly that most relevant to the theme of this chapter is Nancy Kass's (2001) framework for public health interventions. This consists of six questions to ask of a proposed public health programme as follows:

1. What are the public health goals of the proposed programme?
2. How effective is the programme in achieving its goals?
3. What are the known or potential burdens of the programme?
4. Can the burdens be minimised? Are there alternative approaches?
5. Is the programme implemented fairly?
6. How can the benefits and burdens of a programme be fairly balanced?

I think that Kass's approach has a number of positive features that can help anyone interested in formulating frameworks in the future. For example, this framework is grounded on a specific and focused problem (should I introduce a particular public health programme or not?). It provides clear guidance about how the framework is to function and when it is to be used. For example, the structure of the framework is an ordered series of questions (and we are explicitly told to start with question 1 and work down the list). This kind of assistance with what we might call the 'working methods' of a framework is surprisingly rare. Such explicit guidance is essential because, without it, it is perfectly possible to read the content of a framework in a number of different ways. For example, we need to know whether the values or principles are supposed to be of equal value, or whether there is some ordered priority given to them.

However, I also think we can learn from some potential problems with this particular framework, and use this experience to reflect on frameworks in general. Here I will focus on just one of these issues, relating to the way that a particular set of assumptions are at work in the background of this framework. Kass holds that a framework or code for public health must be distinct from those presented and used in clinical medicine, and she characterises this as a need to include what she calls positive as well as negative rights. However, her apparent endorsement of a theoretical expansion to respond to the requirements of public health practice is, I think, in the end illusory. In short, the discussion in the article makes quite clear that the dominant theoretical perspective at work in this framework remains a pretty traditional liberal theory, focused on the value of non-interference. On this approach, we ought to have the freedom to do anything we want unless there is a justifiable reason to restrict that choice. The range of reasons for such a justification is a narrow one (for example, potential harm to others, lack of information, incompetence and so on). The operation of this dominant assumption (despite the claimed expansion) can be seen, for example, in the following quote: "[p]rograms that are coercive should be kept to a minimum, should never be implemented when a less restrictive program would achieve comparable goals, and should be implemented only in the face of clear public health need and good data demonstrating effectiveness" (p 1781). However, this ignores the fact that very often public health authorities are required to act in a situation with limited information. For example, when faced by a novel infectious disease threat with apparent high risk of a deadly outcome, it seems reasonable to prioritise harm prevention (even if it involves a degree of coercion) over individual liberty. Or, to take another example, where a public health threat can be reduced more efficiently and quickly using more coercive means, it should at least be open to debate whether the costs in terms of reduced liberty might not be worth paying as a means of attaining the end more quickly. So my concern is that this framework operates with a dominant (but highly contestable) assumption, one that presents public health as a *problem*, in the sense that pursuing public health ends will inevitably infringe on individual liberties, and the role of this framework becomes one of merely establishing the legitimate limits to personal freedom. Of course, personal freedom is important and ought to be protected. My point is not to deny this, but rather to emphasise that there are many other values that are relevant and (especially in the absence of an argument to this effect) we have no good reason, in formulating public health policy (or a framework for such), always to prioritise liberty. If we are formulating a general framework for public health, then what we need is a framework that truly captures the aims and nature of public health and the fact that such interventions often require a collective rather than merely individual mode of delivery. Such a framework will make it clear that there are multiple equal values that need to be weighed against each other in response to the particular situation. There ought to be no presumption that any particular value (be it liberty or harm prevention) always takes priority.

So, in conclusion of this section, what have we learnt about frameworks? First, a framework is a pragmatic device designed to aid decision making. It 'frames' a response to an issue and aids deliberation in producing an answer, through making relevant values, principles or issues explicit. In addition, the use of a framework allows a certain detachment from potentially controversial theoretical issues (allowing a pragmatic postponement of discussions about justificatory issues). Second, we have no good reason to think of a framework as supplying all of the answers. Frameworks are essentially provisional and heuristic in nature. Nor should frameworks be taken too seriously, in the sense that they are really a kind of rough shorthand and should not be treated as the last word on any topic. We must take care not to be blinded to the real complexity of the circumstances under consideration or to think that the deliberations aided by a framework will result in an end to future discussion. The problem to be addressed ought to drive the framework, rather than the other way round. We have no reason to think that a framework for one area ought to be applied in another, nor should we think of a framework as something we can deductively apply to the facts. It is only a guide. We still need judgement and to take responsibility for the resultant action suggested by the framework. Third, the framework must adequately capture as many of the relevant values as possible; it must explain how the different values relate to each other; and how the framework is to be applied. Do all values have equal weight? If some have greater value than others, why is this, and how do conflicts between the different types of values get resolved? Producing a useful and pragmatic aid to deliberation requires more than the mere listing of elements, issues or principles: any adequate framework needs to make clear how it is to be used.

Theories and assumptions: individual liberty in public health ethics

In this section I move away from a discussion of frameworks and begin to explore the implications of what I take to be the dominating theoretical assumption behind much contemporary public health ethics. This assumption can be seen in the discussion at the core of a number of the chapters in this volume (including Datta and Kessel (Chapter Seven); Hann and Peckham (Chapters Seven and Nine); Sutton and Upshur (Chapter Eleven); and Almark et al (Chapter Five)). In this section I outline its nature and say a little about why I think it is mistaken.[15] The assumption that I am talking about is the conceptualisation of public health ethics as being *about* a real or potential conflict between the individual on the one side and the state, government or society on the other. I suggest that this way of framing these discussions reflects the dominance of a narrow and thin version of liberal political theory. This assumption pushes us to see individual freedom, liberty or autonomy (they tend to all be used as if they were synonymous) as the relevant baseline value to be protected unless there are 'good reasons' not to do so (for example, an act will result in harm to others). This approach involves a commitment to the necessary prioritising of one particular value: individual freedom. It is no surprise, therefore, given the aims of public health and its interest in protecting and promoting health at the population level, that much routine public health activity is seen as problematic because it, allegedly, ignores or sacrifices individuals and their interests for the good of society. This way of framing the discussion is so automatic and prevalent that even critics of individualistic liberalism tend to shape their discussion in these terms (Cribb, Chapter Two), and others explicitly embrace and defend it (Holland, Chapter Three).[16]

This way of conceptualising public health ethics is almost ubiquitous. However, as Holland (Chapter Three) gives the most detailed defence of this approach in this volume, I will discuss his views in some detail. The most common way of framing the discussion is in terms of a need to balance or weigh population and individual interests. However, Holland prefers to picture things in terms of what he calls a "problematic triad" (p 33). He sees the crucial tension as being between individuals and populations – or the "rights and freedoms of individuals" and "the need to protect and promote the health of the population" (p 33) – with government (presumably at the apex of the triad) playing a balancing or arbitrating role between the other two. He then goes on to claim that two political theories, liberalism and utilitarianism, map onto the tension between the individual (liberalism) and population (utilitarianism). I know this is supposed to be just a rough account, but it seems to me to be an odd way to characterise public health ethics. For example, at one point he says "Public health is a utilitarian endeavour in that the whole point of public health is to make the world a better place by implementing policies that protect and improve the health of populations" (p 41). Of course, there is a sense in which this is true, as many aspects of public health policy could be supported by utilitarianism (and historically perhaps no moral theory has had a more practical positive impact upon public health, through the work of the 19th-century reformers). However, framing the discussion in this way encourages us to forget that other moral and political perspectives could also support such policies.[17] Unless there is some necessary link between supporting public health and a commitment to utilitarianism (which there isn't), I think it is unhelpful to define things in these terms.

Although the official story is one of a triad in tension, it does not take long for us to see that Holland actually sees the individual as being the crucial and privileged element in the triad (and so makes evident his commitment to a particular variant of liberalism: that is, liberalism as non-interference). For example, in support of this idea he claims that we ought to incorporate Kant's second formulation of the categorical imperative into public health ethics, "because of the danger inherent in public health's population perspective of using individuals as means to achieving public health goals" (p 42).[18] This exposes the key assumption that I want to point out and discuss in this section. However, perhaps it is worth just briefly mentioning that if anyone wants to develop a Kantian form of public health ethics, I think it is far from obvious that it will be antithetical to public health in the way presumed here. I will give just two reasons for this view. First, the third formulation of the categorical imperative is phrased in terms of the individual developing within a community context. For Kant, it seems that the recognition of personhood, individuality and value is something to be achieved *within* a community, and not something to be seen as *antithetical* to it. Second, it should not be forgotten that Kantian autonomy is about rational autonomy (linking free action with moral responsibility). This is a long way from the 'Millian' story of autonomy as the mere satisfaction of desires or choices that dominates contemporary bioethics (O'Neill, 2003). Indeed, Kantian rational autonomy might be thought to be best pursued in the context of a strong community with strong public health. Leaving Kant to one side, I think this general approach of seeing the individual and population in essential tension and then tending to see the latter as a threat to the former is at the heart of the problem of contemporary public health ethics. However, nothing requires us to see things in terms of an essential conflict between the individual and population, and we certainly have no good reason to then place this at the core of public health policy and practice (and therefore public health ethics). This way of framing things gets it wrong for four main reasons.

First, the implicit model of social relations within this approach ought to be questioned. Why must we think of any individual as if they could be detached from society or their community? Does it even make sense to think in these terms? Even if making the distinction is coherent (and I'm not sure it is), why must we necessarily think of the individual and society as being in conflict with one another (for of course every individual is also a part of a society)? If we think of public health practice and policy, it is actually surprisingly difficult to think of examples where an individual is genuinely 'sacrificed' for the greater good of society. The only cases that seem to fit this extreme scenario involve situations where an individual might have a highly infectious disease that could be a threat to a population (say, a haemorrhagic fever virus). While such an individual might be subject to isolation due to the threat to others, there is no reason to believe that they would not be treated for their disease or (if the situation were sufficiently grave) offered palliative care.[19] We ought not to forget that many benefits derive from our participation as individuals within a society. Only the wildest advocates of libertarianism will want to dismiss them. Such a view is certainly incredible, given the fact that most people can clearly see the benefits of a non-minimal state (such as an education system, clean water and sanitation, an accessible healthcare system, and so on). It often seems to be forgotten that most of the time (at least in the developed world) the government proposing a public health intervention is democratically elected and accountable to the people. State action need not be either arbitrary or unjustifiable and, of course, no politician will want to run too far ahead of what voters find acceptable. Public health departments are, in turn, accountable to government, and ultimately, the electorate.

Second, as mentioned in the discussion of frameworks, while liberty is an important value, it can surely be trumped or overridden by other values at least on some occasions, for example, where there is harm to others (smoking bans in public places or workplaces); harm to vulnerable groups (smoking ban in cars when children are present); the promotion of better water quality and the environment (ban on the domestic use of weed killers and lawn feed); or protection of the public from possible contaminants and pathogens (food and restaurant inspections and compulsory pasteurisation of milk). It is important to see that there may be strong objections in these cases if government decides to do nothing. Foreseeable harm may result from giving priority to liberty. I think it makes more sense to see these debates as being competitions between equal values, rather than seeing liberty as the default value unless it is 'overruled' by some other reason. So it is important to see that I am not arguing in favour of *prioritising* an alternative value. Health, for example, should not be seen as the only relevant value, or as that which is always the most important. Rather, I want to suggest that all relevant values (and there are many) are of equal weight and can be traded against each other. Sometimes liberty will win out, and other times other values. Such equal plural values, then, have structural similarities to prima facie obligations (Dawson and Garrard, 2006).

Third, public health is about the protection and promotion of population health (Verweij and Dawson, 2007). It is often just assumed that population health is the mere aggregation of the health of all the relevant individuals, but this is not the case. To give just one example, a population with fewer cases of alcohol-related disease has better public health. If we think this is true, we ought not merely to focus on trying to provide information to individuals or change the behaviour of individuals. This is because we know that there is a complex interactive relationship between individual and population health. For example, the drinking culture of a society will influence the number of 'problem drinkers'. The degree of alcohol regulation in a given society is due to societal and cultural attitudes, and this changes individual behaviour and so impacts on individual health through population-level interventions (Rose, 1992). In addition, we should not forget that public health interventions can be expressive of the kind of society we want to live in. They can actually instantiate important values such as solidarity, the fact that we care about each other and that we want to improve the place where *we* live.[20]

Fourth, public health aims to improve population health, but it often does so, and sometimes can only do so, through collective interventions (Verweij and Dawson, 2007). For example, if we are interested in reducing health inequalities in society, and know something of the socio-economic determinants of health, the kinds of interventions that will be appropriate cannot just be focused on individuals because an individual's health is at least partly the result of the way that each individual relates to others in that society. The state can do all kinds of things to assure the conditions for health in a way that individuals alone cannot, for example, through the provision of infrastructure for a healthy life (such as cycle lanes, parks, footpaths); quality control (for example, food inspection and regulation, pasteurisation of milk, provision of clean water and sanitation); legislation to reduce inequalities and tackle health problems such as obesity (for example, to increase exercise programmes in schools); and the regulation of behaviour through taxation (for example, high taxation on tobacco, or providing tax breaks for healthy behaviours and so on).

My main point is that the presumption in favour of liberty is something that we can choose to adopt if we wish, but we don't have to do so. We have a choice that many do not seem to be aware of. The choice to prioritise liberty involves a way of framing the issues and a set of commitments that we need not accept. Indeed, if we are sympathetic to the aims of public health, there is a lot to be said for critiquing and then rejecting this dominating presumption – especially as the result is a readiness to criticise the 'nanny state' and adopt a minimalism about the aims of public policy. I think that we need to develop a more mature language to use in our discussion about public policy and public health; one that does not phrase things in terms of 'bans' or just assume that 'banning' something is always a bad thing. Individual freedom is a vital component of living well, but many other actions can also promote the good life. Some of these options require a sacrifice of liberty, but this can be worth it. Public health, given its aims to promote and protect health, and the fact that many collective interventions are essential to attain that end, is an example of where such a mature public policy would be welcome.

Conclusions

In this chapter I have argued that we need to take care to distinguish theories, frameworks and models and that the key to doing so is through noting the three different roles that they may have. I have argued that frameworks are a useful means to draw the more theoretical and practical together, but have suggested the need for more care in their development, in terms of their focus, internal consistency and the way they are to be used. I have also argued that we need to evaluate critically the hidden assumptions not only in our theoretical discussions about public health ethics but also when we think about the justification of policy interventions.

Running through this whole chapter is an alternative way of conceptualising public health ethics, one that builds out from public health practice. This approach consists in adopting a number of important but equal moral values focused on attaining the ends of public health. No single value, whether it is liberty, harm reduction or anything else, ought to have automatic priority over others. This means that public health ethics cannot simply apply the approach commonly adopted in much contemporary medical ethics, but this does not necessarily mean that public health ethics ought to be a separate domain. It may or may not be the case that we can have a unified theory for both medical and public health ethics: that remains to be seen. However, I remain confident that thinking about public health, and public health ethics, will actually lead to the development of a richer and more sophisticated version of medical ethics in the future.

Notes

[1] Thanks to Ross Upshur and Barb Secker for discussion of an earlier version of this chapter.

[2] Cribb (Chapter Two) also argues for the need for an interdisciplinary and practice-relevant conversation at the core of public health ethics.

[3] See Krieger (2008) for discussion of the way that diagrams or representations in general can shape our comprehension of issues in public health (sometimes aiding, sometimes confusing). The same is often true of metaphors. A metaphor should be used to aid our understanding, not be a substitute for it. The metaphors used in explanations, in my view, often require much more explication than they generally receive.

[4] An example of confusion about these different roles can be found in the Nuffield Council on Bioethics' report on public health ethics (2007). When it talks of its preferred "framework" (ch 2) it in fact produces something that it calls "the stewardship model" (pp 25–6). The proposed "model" is really a framework (although it is a rather odd mixture of highly normative aims and constraints that programmes "should" abide by (p 26)). For some other problems with the Nuffield approach see Dawson and Verweij (2008).

[5] This role-driven approach will also reinforce the importance of the relevance of different disciplines in the pursuit of these different ends. Philosophers may be most interested in the development of theory, but they will also be interested in the other concepts. Social scientists may be most interested in the production of models, but they will have something to say about the other tasks too, and so on.

[6] See, in particular, Daniels (1996) for discussion of reflective equilibrium.

[7] This is a complex issue, and this is not the place to discuss the problems with coherentist epistemologies, but briefly, I think coherence among a set of beliefs is too easy to achieve without any of the component beliefs actually being true.

[8] I explore what this means for public health ethics in much more detail in Dawson (2009).

[9] However, in my proposed taxonomy such uses are not so close to the core of the concept of a framework. Such 'frameworks' are closer either to a theory (because they are justificatory) or a model (as they explain the decisions made).

[10] Kass (2001) talks about the research ethics principles deriving from the Belmont Report, the four principles, an ethics of care, casuistry and virtue-based ethics as though they were all frameworks (p 1777). I think such loose talk is unhelpful. The four principles and Belmont may just about count as frameworks; but casuistry is more of a method; an ethics of care is difficult to classify, as the term covers such a diverse range of things; and surely virtue ethics is a paradigm case of a normative theory.

[11] Again, I think the Nuffield Council on Bioethics' (2007) stewardship model or framework counts as a good example of such a confused approach.

[12] Kass also claims that we live in "a morally pluralistic society, and it is inevitable that moral appeals will conflict" (2001, p 1777) and, according to her, this provides a reason why we need frameworks to help decision making.

[13] There are many problems in the adoption of procedural values. All I will note here is that procedural values cannot be used to *replace* substantive values in the construction of frameworks, so they cannot be used as a means to sidestep any disagreement over substantive values.

[14] See, for example, Verweij and Dawson (2004) for a suggested framework for policy making in relation to mass preventive vaccination programmes.

[15] I say much more about the reasons why I think it is mistaken in other places; see, especially, Dawson (2009).

[16] Something like this view also seems to be one of the influences on the complaint about 'medicalisation' in medicine and public health (Zola, 1972; Fitzpatrick, 2001).

[17] It is also, perhaps, worth pointing out that even if we wish to stick to the 19th century, many reformers were both liberals and utilitarians.

[18] Apparently dropping Kant's "*mere* means".

[19] So, it seems to me that it is hard to think of any scenario outside of a thought experiment-type objection to consequentialism, where an individual will be 'used as a means' in the relevant way for this conceptualisation to make any sense.

[20] It is a common tactic for opponents of government regulation to claim that 'bans' do not or will not work. However, even if we leave to one side the empirical facts about whether such claims are true, we should not forget the symbolic value that many such policies can have. In addition, while a public health intervention may result *from* a shift in attitudes, it may also contribute to *creating* or *reinforcing* such changes. Such changes can be seen, for example, in relation to attitudes towards smoking.

References

Childress, J.F, Faden, R.R., Gaare, R.D., Gostin, L.O., Kahn, J., Bonnie, R.J., Kass, N.E., Mastroianni, A.C., Moreno, J.D. and Nieburg, P. (2002) 'Public health ethics: mapping the terrain', *The Journal of Law, Medicine & Ethics*, vol 30, no 2, pp 170–8.

Daniels, N. (1996) *Justice and justification: Reflective equilibrium in theory and practice*, Cambridge: Cambridge University Press.

Dawson, A. (2009) 'Resetting the parameters: public health as the foundation for public health ethics', in A. Dawson (ed) *Public health ethics: Key concepts and issues in policy and practice*, Cambridge: Cambridge University Press.

Dawson, A. and Garrard, E. (2006) 'In defence of moral imperialism: four equal and universal prima facie duties', *Journal of Medical Ethics*, vol 32, no 4, pp 200–4.

Dawson, A. and Verweij, M. (2008) 'The steward of the Millian state', *Public Health Ethics*, vol 1, no 3, pp 193–5.

Fitzpatrick, M. (2001) *The tyranny of health: Doctors and the regulation of lifestyle*, London: Routledge.

Giacomini, M., Kenny, N. and DeJean, D. (2009) 'Ethics frameworks in Canadian health policies: Foundation, scaffolding, or window dressing?', *Health Policy*, vol 89, pp 58–71.

Kass, N. (2001) 'An ethics framework for public health', *American Journal of Public Health*, vol 91, no 11, pp 1776–82.

Krieger, N. (2008) 'Ladders, pyramids and champagne: the iconography of health inequities', *Journal of Epidemiology and Community Health*, vol 62, pp 1098–104.

Nuffield Council on Bioethics (2007) *Public health: Ethical issues*, London: Nuffield Council on Bioethics.

O'Neill, O. (2003) 'Autonomy: the emperor's new clothes', *Proceedings of the Aristotelian Society, Supplementary Volume*, vol 77, pp 1–21.

Rose, G. (1992) *The strategy of preventive medicine*, Oxford: Oxford University Press.

Verweij, M. and Dawson, A. (2004) 'Ethical principles for collective immunisation programmes', *Vaccine*, vol 22, pp 3122–6.

Verweij, M. and Dawson, A. (2007) 'The meaning of "public" in "public health"', in A. Dawson and M. Verweij (eds) *Ethics, prevention and public health*, Oxford: Oxford University Press.

Zola, I.K. (1972) 'Medicine as an institution of social control', *Sociological Review*, vol 20, pp 487–504.

THIRTEEN

Conclusion: taking forward the debate

Stephen Peckham and Alison Hann

Every day public health practitioners are faced by many dilemmas in their practice. The discussions in the chapters in this book have addressed some of the old and new areas of ethical debate in public health. Developing coherent and effective health promotion messages is clearly important, as is thinking about how we should respond to new technologies such as new vaccines, and potential public health threats such as pandemic flu and resistant strains of TB. There are also difficult debates about the nature of evidence in public health and the extent to which evidence can and even should be the main guide for policy and practice. Public health has been described as 'social action' and, therefore, governed by different paradigms from clinical medecine, and evidence should consequently play a different role. What is certain and clearly described by the chapters of this book is that ethics should be a primary concern of public health. Angus Dawson argued in Chapter Twelve that public health ethics needs to be built up from public health practice. This is a central theme of the book.

Much revolves around the role of government, as it sets the context within which public health policies and practice are developed and implemented. Steve Holland argued in his chapter that it is important to examine the legitimate circumstances of public health action by governments in relation to the individual and the wider community. This is a view echoed by the Nuffield Council on Bioethics, which supported the concept of the 'stewardship role' of government. Stewardship is defined as the social contract between government and its people, whereby government processes are performed in trust for the people and founded on principles of ethics as well as efficiency (Saltman and Ferroussier-Davis, 2000). The very nature of stewardship implies a stronger activist role by government to ensure that ethically sound and efficient policy is formulated and delivered for the greatest good. Stewardship implies that governments have the responsibility not only to use public funds in a responsible manner, but also to invest these in ways that address suffering among its poorest people and reduce inequality among its citizens. This reflects Steve Holland's arguments in Chapter Three about the relationship between individuals, communities and the state. But Alan Cribb's arguments (Chapter Two) are also central to developing this concept. As Angus Dawson argues in Chapter Twelve, stewardship is not, in itself, a framework, but provides a statement about the nature and role of governments. Such a concept requires a broader understanding of the nature of society and the relationship between governing and society, and this suggests a somewhat different framework for an ethical approach to public health that rests in the nature of society itself.

Given the complexities of health issues, the relationships between individuals, and the relationships between individuals and government, it is clear that in future ethical issues in public health will be even more central than they are now. The way we, as a society, view public health problems, individual liberty, community relationships and the role of government continues to change. This is reflected in the subject matter of the chapters in this book. Immunisation, pandemics, obesity and smoking are key public health issues subject to health policy and practice. Likewise health promotion, health protection and the role of health workers are topics that are neither value-neutral nor free from controversy. In the opening chapter we argued that, in future, there will be more and more ways to monitor people, more public awareness of threats to public health, and an awareness that there are ethical and possibly legal (such as enforced quarantine) difficulties with the distribution of harms and benefits. Balancing the rights and responsibilities of individuals and wider populations is becoming more complex. There is clearly a need to develop this debate and we hope that this book will play a role in opening out a discussion of public health ethics into the public health practice arena. The chapters in the last section of the book set out some of the parameters of this debate.

In the previous chapter, Angus Dawson argued that adherence to specific or rigid ethical frameworks is not appropriate for the application of ethics in public health practice. Yet we do need some guidance or way to consider ethical practice. This search for an ethical framework can be seen in the deliberations of the Nuffield Council on Bioethics' working party report on public health ethics (Nuffield Council on Bioethics, 2007). The report highlights the complexities of balancing different aspects of harm, benefit, risk, autonomy and choice. It advocates a precautionary approach to public health interventions.

The concept of a precautionary principle is one that has wide acceptance within public health circles. However, while there is acceptance of the principle it is not clear when and how that principle should be used. As the Nuffield Council report (2007) states: "The precise meaning of the principle has been the subject of intense debates … in applying the precautionary principle it is important to recognise that it is not a single inflexible rule, but a way of applying a set of interacting criteria to a given situation" (p 35). The Council adopts what it calls a precautionary approach, which is seen as reflecting the concept of a set of criteria, and reflects the dynamic nature of their application. It refers to the European Commission's five elements:

- scientific assessment of risk, acknowledging uncertainties and updated in the light of new evidence
- fairness and consistency
- consideration of costs and benefits of actions
- transparency
- proportionality.

While these elements are apparently self-evident and provide a clear framework, problems occur in their application and interpretation. There are two key elements where particular problems can occur. The first is in terms of evidence of effect, and the other relates to the concept of proportionality. On the one hand, evidence of benefit and/or harm may not be conclusive. There is often scientific debate about the nature or extent of the benefits and harms of public health interventions. Allmark et al, in Chapter Five of this volume, demonstrate, for example, how what may appear to be a harmless intervention – health education on giving up smoking – may in fact cause harm because messages are not clarified, despite the approach seemingly being one that should not result in harm, but only benefit. Clearly, public health professionals and policy makers should ensure that any intervention is supported by the best evidence, although the level and quality of the evidence will be contingent on the level of risk. As the Rio Declaration states: "Where there are threats of serious or irreversible damage, lack of full scientific certainty shall not be used as a reason for postponing cost-effective measures to prevent environmental degradation" (Rio Declaration on the Environment, 1992). Kriebel and Tickner (2001) argue that, while the Rio Declaration was addressing environmental concerns, the principle applies equally to public health actions. But as Holland (2007) argues, "a major problem with the [precautionary principle] in public health is that it permits overly intrusive, Draconian interventions" (p 32).

In some cases, however, there may be a lack of evidence as to harm. As the Nuffield Council questioned, does the lack of evidence about harm mean that something is not harmful? In health this is a key question, and is dependent on whether or not evidence has been gathered and made public. Healthcare evidence is particularly susceptible to bias, due to non-published results orcommercial pressures (such as in relation to tobacco, use of statins). In addition, in some cases evidence is not clear and is contested. The Nuffield Council's approach to this is to have recourse to procedural approaches to dealing with public health action, such as in relation to water fluoridation, where it refers to the need for local democratic involvement. But, as Dawson remarks in Chapter Twelve in relation to the process approach inherent in Kass's (2001) framework or that proposed by Giacomini et al (2009), such an approach does not always provide a reasonable basis for ethical action. In summary, Dawson argues that public health practitioners need to adopt "a number of important but equal moral values focused on attaining the ends of public health. No single value, whether it is liberty, harm reduction or anything else, ought to have automatic priority over others. This means that public health ethics cannot simply apply the approach commonly adopted in much contemporary medical ethics" (pp 205-6).

But public health action and the roles and actions of professionals are guided by a range of criteria, including the values of professional practice developed through public health training, public health policy that sets out goals and targets for public health, and institutional structures and processes. These both are autonomous frames for action and also serve to structure and reinforce particular sets of criteria. The recent development of the Quality Outcomes Framework (QOF) in the UK, which rewards GPs for undertaking certain measurements such as blood pressure and cholesterol levels, is an example of how such criteria are institutionalised in practice through financial reward. For example, while the current guidance on 'Lipid modification' issued by the National Institute for Health and Clinical Excellence suggests that, in order to lower the risk of cardiovascular disease patients should be offered life-style advice and be advised to eat a low (saturated) fat diet, eating five portions of fruit per day (another area where there is little supportive evidence of effectiveness), the pressure to ensure that patients' cholesterol levels are lowered has led to a steady increase in the use of statins, despite the poor evidence of effect in general use.

Since the introduction of QOF, GPs have focused attention on maximising their QOF points, and the evidence demonstrates that this has led to high levels of success in this, with some small variations for practice size and socio-economic context (with practices serving smaller and less deprived populations performing better) (McDonald et al, 2007). While this can be seen as an achievement, there is some evidence that the quality of care in incentivised areas such as coronary heart disease had been increasing anyway (Campbell et al, 2007). One key aspect of incentives is that practices ensure that they reach their threshold payment levels. Harrison and Smith (2004) have argued that financial incentives can lead to adverse behaviour changes, leading to goal misplacement in which rule following becomes the means to the end). Thus, the object becomes achieving the threshold target, and lowering serum cholesterol levels rather than focusing on maximising patient care and outcomes. This is but one small way in which practitioners who are not trained public health practitioners undertake public health action framed by policy, guidance and incentives. With the increasing push towards a public health workforce that encapsulates the whole of the public, private and third sectors, the need for clear guidance built on sound ethical principles becomes even more important.

Frameworks and codes

But where does this leave the practitioner? Rather than developing frameworks and codes of practice for public health ethics, our aim in this book has been to present ethical problems within a practice and policy context. Some authors have put forward ways of approaching such ethical dilemmas, but it has not been our intention to develop an ethical framework. This has been done by other authors but, as the Nuffield Council on Bioethics' report demonstrates, it is the processes of applying ethics to practice and policy that remain a key problem. But authors in this book caution us against drawing ethics only from a practice base or from a theoretical standpoint. We are perhaps left, then, with an approach that brings both these domains together. However, public health practice, as Holland reminds us, takes place within a political context. In addition, public health action is shaped by many forces, changing constantly in response to policy shifts, professionalisation, financial regimes and incentives, local contexts and, as shown in this book, by misconceptions and strongly held beliefs (and competing moral and cultural contexts). Public health ethics and public health practice exist, therefore, very much within a contested space: their very nature, however, may threaten the ability of public health to protect and improve health.

To develop a public health ethics we need to create internal and external coherence regarding its sources and norms, and deliver an identifiable corpus of ethical principles that is robust enough to inform practice in changing and difficult environments. The lack of such clarity presents a radical challenge to public health and the risk that the field may lose direction or influence, and has resulted in parallel ethical discourses which can be impossible to dialogue.

As Dawson has commented in Chapter Twelve, while a NHS medical-ethics dominant reading of public health has never been the only reading of public health ethics, this reading is increasingly challenged by the readings from voluntary and community sectors, public policy and other professions. A medical-ethics reading cannot be the dominant discourse for the future if public health ethics is successfully to complete the project of developing sufficient coherence to live in this contested space.

Next steps

Currently in the UK there is little training for public health workers on ethical issues. The Faculty of Public Health addresses only the ethics of personal conduct within the current professional framework. There is in fact little reference to ethics within the public health training framework for practitioners. In 2003 guidelines for health protection, reference is made to the need for training in public health so as to ensure that all trainees understand professional principles, including confidentiality *and ethics*. However, a search for references to ethics on the Faculty's website or in its publications focuses mainly on acting ethically or in reference to research ethics. In the US there is an increasing emphasis on training public health practitioners about ethics, and public health ethics is now a key element of postgraduate education in public health in the major schools of public health. Similarly in Canada, there is a growing interest in public health ethics and in incorporating ethics training into education programmes. It is clear that, if public health practice is to develop in the UK, it is essential for training in ethics to become an integral part of the public health training programme. If we are to aspire to linking ethics and ethical practice, then those practising public health need to be able to draw on a substantive knowledge base.

This book started with a conference that brought together public health practitioners, ethicists and social scientists, and it is perhaps fitting that we should end with a number of key points made at the conference. Debates there highlighted a number of issues that were considered important to ensure that ethical considerations were incorporated into future developments for public health policy and practice and into public health training. Conference participants were particularly keen that public health professional organisations responsible for developing public health curricula, such as the Faculty of Public Health, should incorporate ethics as a key part of training and continuing professional development (CPD) activity. Examples of existing training were given from the West Midlands and from some Masters degree courses, but ethics is not a core requirement in public health training. While the value of CPD training was widely acknowledged, there was a clear call for education agencies and those training public health professionals to incorporate ethics into their educational programmes. This would be strengthened by ethics being made part of the core standards for public health practice.

But the notion of core standards needs to go beyond the registered public health professional. Delegates were keen to see ethical decision making integrated into the practice of public health professionals and of the wider public health workforce. Whatever interventions are undertaken need to be done across a range of levels, working with people on how they acquire ethical and critical thinking and use it in practice. These levels include policy makers and public health specialists, and also a host of other agencies (such as environmental health, local authority, voluntary sector, nursing, health visitors and so on). While some work is already being undertaken in this area through academic subject networks and also locally in Masters in Public Health programmes it needs to be more widespread and to be recognised as a key skill. Other key activities that need to be pursued in the immediate future if public health practitioners are to be equipped to deal with increasingly complex public health problems include developing a framework for public health ethics; running workshops along the lines of those already developed by the Critical Appraisal Skills Programme that introduce ethical analysis to practitioners and board members; developing training packages for executives and non-executives in local NHS organisations – such as Primary Care Trusts, Local Health Boards, Community Health Partnerships and health authorities; developing educational models for teaching public health ethics; working with the Faculty of Public Health and others; and providing a system of emergency ethical support for practitioners who are faced with key ethical dilemmas in their everyday practice. Public health ethics is a developing field of practice and study. However, true understanding and ethical practice will only come about as practitioners and others responsible for public health practice engage with ethical ideas and frameworks to reach an ethics of public health practice.

References

Campbell, S., Reeves, D., Kontopantelis, E., Middleton, E., Sibbald, B. and Roland, M. (2007) 'Quality of primary care in England with the introduction of pay for performance', *New England Journal of Medicine*, vol 357, no 2, pp 181–90.

Giacomini, M., Kenny, N. and DeJean, D. (2009) 'Ethics frameworks in Canadian health policies: foundation, scaffolding, or window dressing?', *Health Policy*, vol 89, pp 58–71.

Harrison, S. and Smith, C. (2004) 'Trust and moral motivation: redundant resources in health and social care?', *Policy & Politics*, vol 32, no 3, pp 371–86.

Holland, S. (2007) *Public health ethics*, Cambridge: Polity Press.

Kass, N.E. (2001) 'An ethics framework for public health', *Public Health Matters*, vol 91, no 11, pp 1776-82.

Kriebel, D. and Tickner, J. (2001) 'Reenergizing public health through precaution', *American Journal of Public Health*, vol 91, pp 1351–5.

McDonald, R., Harrison, S., Checkland, K., Campbell, S. and Roland, R. (2007) 'Impact of financial incentives on clinical autonomy and internal motivation in primary care: an ethnographic study', *British Medical Journal*, vol 334, pp 1357–60.

Nuffield Council on Bioethics (2007) *Public health ethics*, London: Nuffield Council on Bioethics.

Rio Declaration on Environment and Development (1992). Available at www.igc.org/habitat/agenda21/rio-dec.html.

Saltman, R.B. and Ferroussier-Davis, O. (2000) 'The concept of stewardship in health policy', *Bulletin of the World Health Organization*, vol 78, no 6, pp 732–9.

Index

Page references for notes are followed by n